Arteriovenous Fistula Management

Nurten Ozen · Clemente Neves Sousa · Paulo Teles

Arteriovenous Fistula Management

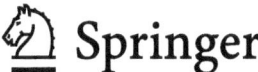

Editors
Nurten Ozen
Faculty of Nursing
Department of Internal Medicine Nursing
Istanbul University
Istanbul, Turkey

Paulo Teles
School of Economics
University of Porto
Porto, Portugal

Clemente Neves Sousa
Nursing School of University of Porto
Porto, Portugal

ISBN 978-3-032-04770-0   ISBN 978-3-032-04771-7   (eBook)
https://doi.org/10.1007/978-3-032-04771-7

© The Editor(s) (if applicable) and The Author(s), under exclusive license to Springer Nature Switzerland AG 2025

This work is subject to copyright. All rights are solely and exclusively licensed by the Publisher, whether the whole or part of the material is concerned, specifically the rights of translation, reprinting, reuse of illustrations, recitation, broadcasting, reproduction on microfilms or in any other physical way, and transmission or information storage and retrieval, electronic adaptation, computer software, or by similar or dissimilar methodology now known or hereafter developed.
The use of general descriptive names, registered names, trademarks, service marks, etc. in this publication does not imply, even in the absence of a specific statement, that such names are exempt from the relevant protective laws and regulations and therefore free for general use.
The publisher, the authors and the editors are safe to assume that the advice and information in this book are believed to be true and accurate at the date of publication. Neither the publisher nor the authors or the editors give a warranty, expressed or implied, with respect to the material contained herein or for any errors or omissions that may have been made. The publisher remains neutral with regard to jurisdictional claims in published maps and institutional affiliations.

This Springer imprint is published by the registered company Springer Nature Switzerland AG
The registered company address is: Gewerbestrasse 11, 6330 Cham, Switzerland

If disposing of this product, please recycle the paper.

Preface

End-stage renal disease is considered a public health problem in many Western countries, not only because of its social, personal and family impact but also because of the economic implications for healthcare systems. Haemodialysis is one of the most widely used treatment methods worldwide among renal replacement therapies. Patients undergo significant changes from the moment they start haemodialysis treatment, with the need for a vascular access and the need to care for the access throughout the treatment process.

The arteriovenous fistula is considered the "ideal access" for haemodialysis patients and is essential not only for carrying out the treatment but also for maintaining a satisfactory quality of life. The book "*Arteriovenous Fistula Management: A Guide to Care Integration*" is the result of many years of practice, research and dedication to the care of haemodialysis patients with arteriovenous fistulas.

We recognise that nephrology nurses play a crucial role in the management of vascular accesses, especially arteriovenous fistulas, from their creation to their monitoring and maintenance, as well as in training patients about the care needed to preserve them. However, despite the importance of this topic, professionals are faced with gaps in access to practical, up-to-date and specific materials to guide them in their daily practice. This book is designed to fill those gaps, providing a comprehensive and structured guide to help nephrology nurses fulfil their role safely, efficiently and with confidence.

We believe that knowledge gives power and that well-prepared nephrology nurses can transform the experience of care for both the patient and the multi-professional team. We hope that this guide will become a valuable resource in your arsenal of knowledge and a constant reference in your clinical practice.

Finally, we would like to express our deep gratitude to all the nursing professionals who dedicate their efforts to caring for kidney patients on a daily basis.

Best wishes for learning and success.

Porto, Portugal Clemente Neves Sousa
December 2025 Nurten Ozen
Paulo Teles

Introduction

The Arteriovenous Fistula was first described in 1966 by Dr. Michael Brescia, Dr. James Cimino, Dr. Kenneth Appel and Dr. Baruch Hurwich at the Bronx Veterans Affairs Medical Center in New York. The Brescia–Cimino innovation consisted of connecting an artery to a vein in the patient's forearm, creating a connection that allowed for high and continuous blood flow, necessary for haemodialysis sessions. This creation represented a milestone in the history of nephrology and provided more efficient and safe vascular access for haemodialysis.

Even after more than 60 years, the arteriovenous fistula continues to be widely used and recommended as the first choice for vascular access. Several studies show that patients with an operational fistula have a lower risk of infection, thrombosis and vascular access complications associated with hospitalization. From its conception to its ongoing care, arteriovenous fistula requires meticulous attention, technical competence and up-to-date knowledge from healthcare professionals. Nephrologist nurses have a crucial contribution to maintaining functionality and preventing complications that directly impact the quality of life and safety of patients. It also stands out for its proximity to the patient, its ability to early problem detection and its ability to promote the development of fistula self-care behaviours by the patient.

This book is designed to provide a structured approach, combining theory and practice, thus enabling nephrology nurses to have an integrative view on the care of arteriovenous fistulas. The approach was structured to cover everything from basic concepts to more complex situations, promoting progressive learning based on scientific evidence. Chapters have been designed to meet the needs of both nurses and nephrology specialist nurses seeking to gain knowledge on this subject.

The first three chapters address care models associated with the arteriovenous fistula and the anatomy of the vascular network, as well as the physiology of the maturation process. The different types of fistulas are also described.

The fourth chapter describes in detail the physical examination as a simple, practical and non-invasive tool that allows assessing the functionality of the fistula and detecting possible complications.

The complications of the arteriovenous fistula are described in the fifth chapter, highlighting venous stenosis, haemodialysis access-induced distal ischaemia, steal syndrome and high flow access. Aspects related to risk factors, diagnosis or clinical assessment are addressed as well.

The sixth chapter discusses monitoring and surveillance and their importance in detecting complications in order to increase the patency of the arteriovenous fistula.

Cannulation methods of the arteriovenous fistula, as well as models that can assist the nephrologist nurse in making decisions to choose the appropriate cannulation for each patient, are covered in the seventh chapter. Complications that may result from the cannulation of an arteriovenous fistula are addressed in the eighth chapter.

The ninth chapter highlights the importance of ultrasound as an indispensable tool in the evaluation and management of the arteriovenous fistula. Furthermore, the impact of using ultrasound on safe cannulation, monitoring and surveillance of the arteriovenous fistula is discussed. Aspects related to nurse empowerment are also addressed.

Patients with end-stage renal disease must adopt self-care behaviours to preserve the vascular network and prevent complications associated with the arteriovenous fistula such as infection, thrombosis or others. In the tenth chapter, issues concerning arteriovenous self-care are listed from the continuous perspective of care from pre-dialysis to haemodialysis treatment.

This book brings together specific scientific knowledge about the arteriovenous fistula, as well as the authors' clinical experience in caring for patients with this kind of access. We believe this book can contribute to strengthening nursing practice and improving the care provided to haemodialysis-dependent patients. This book can be a source of inspiration and knowledge, helping nephrology nurses to feel more confident and prepared to deal with the challenges of caring for people with arteriovenous fistulas.

Enjoy your reading.

Clemente Neves Sousa
Nurten Ozen
Paulo Teles

Contents

1. **History and Model of Arteriovenous Fistula Care** 1
   Clemente Neves Sousa and Paulo Teles
2. **Creation of an Arteriovenous Fistula** 9
   Clemente Neves Sousa, Nurten Ozen, and António Norton de Matos
3. **Physical Examination of the Arteriovenous Fistula**. 21
   Nurten Ozen and Clemente Neves Sousa
4. **Arteriovenous Fistula Complications** 29
   Nurten Ozen, Clemente Neves Sousa, and Tayfun Eyileten
5. **Monitoring and Surveillance of an Arteriovenous Fistula** 39
   Nurten Ozen and Clemente Neves Sousa
6. **Cannulation Methods for the Arteriovenous Fistula**. 51
   Clemente Neves Sousa, Nurten Ozen, and Paulo Teles
7. **Complications in Arteriovenous Fistula Cannulation** 63
   Nurten Ozen and Clemente Neves Sousa
8. **Ultrasound for the Arteriovenous Fistula**. 71
   Clemente Neves Sousa, Nurten Ozen, Paulo Teles, Tanju Kisbet, and
   Volkan Ozen
9. **Self-care Behaviours with the Arteriovenous Fistula** 81
   Clemente Neves Sousa, Nurten Ozen, and Paulo Teles

Contributors

António Norton de Matos Grupo de Estudos Vasculares (Vascular Access Center), Porto, Portugal

Clemente Neves Sousa Nursing School of University of Porto, Porto, Portugal
RISE – Health, University of Porto, Porto, Portugal

Nurten Ozen Faculty of Nursing, Department of Internal Medicine Nursing, Istanbul University, Istanbul, Turkey

Paulo Teles School of Economics, University of Porto, Porto, Portugal
LIAAD-INESC Porto LA, Porto, Portugal

Tanju Kisbet Prof. Dr. Cemil Tascioglu City Hospital, Department of Radiology, Istanbul, Turkey

Tayfun Eyileten Guven Hospital, Department of Nephrology, Ankara, Turkey

Volkan Ozen Prof. Dr. Cemil Tascioglu City Hospital, Department of Anesthesiology and Reanimation, Istanbul, Turkey

History and Model of Arteriovenous Fistula Care

Clemente Neves Sousa and Paulo Teles

In recent decades, the prevalence and incidence of chronic diseases have increased worldwide. Several factors are associated with that increase, such as population growth, increasing life expectancy and improving economic conditions. Chronic kidney disease (CKD) is a growing problem in developed or developing countries leading to an increase in patients requiring dialysis treatment. In the United States of America (USA), CKD is considered a public health problem with major socioeconomic repercussions for the health system and the society (Jager et al. 2019).

Over 850 million people worldwide suffer from CKD. The overall incidence has increased by 89% in the last three decades (Clementi et al. 2020). The rising incidence of diabetes mellitus, obesity and hypertension has led to the growing number of patients with CKD. The prevalence of end stage renal disease (ESRD) varies across Europe, depending on the country.

Portugal is the country with the highest incidence and prevalence of ESRD in the world, with 235.9 and 1577.9 per million people (pmp) in 2010 and 226.49 and 1661.9 pmp in 2011, respectively (Coelho et al. 2014; Clementi et al. 2020). The lowest incidences in 2003–2016 were reported by South Africa, Ukraine, Belarus, Bangladesh, Russia, Jordan, Peru, Colombia, Iran, Albania and Estonia, ranging from 22 to 85 pmp/year (Thurlow et al. 2021). Statistics show CKD is rising, even if

---

C. N. Sousa (✉)
Nursing School of University of Porto, Porto, Portugal
e-mail: clementesousa@esenf.pt

RISE – Health, University of Porto, Porto, Portugal

P. Teles
School of Economics, University of Porto, Porto, Portugal
e-mail: pteles@fep.up.pt

LIAAD – INESC Porto LA, Porto, Portugal

© The Author(s), under exclusive license to Springer Nature Switzerland AG 2025
N. Ozen et al. (eds.), *Arteriovenous Fistula Management*,
https://doi.org/10.1007/978-3-032-04771-7_1

at different rates, which means that patients need appropriate vascular access in order to undergo haemodialysis treatment. Creation of an arteriovenous fistula (AVF) can be a challenge for the vascular surgeon.

1 History and Epidemiology of the Arteriovenous Fistula

The first AVF was created in 19 February 1965, with side-by-side anastomosis between the radial artery and the cephalic vein at the wrist. Brescia et al. published the article "Chronic hemodialysis using venepuncture and a surgically created arteriovenous fistula" in 1966, after 16 months of experimenting with a radiocephalic AVF (Brescia et al. 1966). In 1976, Dagher et al. published the first article on the use of veins from the deep venous system (basilic vein) in haemodialysis (Dagher et al. 1976). During the 1980s and 1990s, the brachial and femoral veins began to be used in the creation of an AVF.

AVF is the recommended vascular access for haemodialysis treatment by several vascular access guidelines. Japan is one of the countries with the highest prevalence of AVF as vascular access (Sato et al. 2019). According to the Japanese Society of Dialysis Therapy, an AVF was used in 89.7% of cases, a graft arteriovenous in 7.1%, superficialization of the brachial artery in 1.8% and an indwelling catheter in 0.5% in Japan (Fukasawa 2019). Furthermore, an AVF was used in 68% of cases in the USA in 2012–2014, after implementation of the Fistula First Initiative (Sato et al. 2019). The percentage of AVF remained roughly constant in the range of 60%–65% in the USA. However, 68% of AVFs were created in the upper arm and only 32% were formed in the lower arm in the USA in 2016. In contrast, more than 90% of AVFs were created in the lower arm in Japan in 2016 (Sato et al. 2019).

In Europe, the percentage of AVF can range from 59% to 80% of prevalent patients in Germany, Italy, Spain, Sweden and Belgium in 2018 (Fukasawa 2019; Sato et al. 2019). The proportion of AVF is 78% of cases in Portugal in 2019. The percentage of lower arm AVF rearing is in the range 65%–77% in Europe in 2018, which is much lower than in Japan (Bello et al. 2022).

Promoting and encouraging the creation of AVF as an appropriate vascular access for haemodialysis treatment are very important. Nephrologist nurses can contribute to patient awareness and to the development of a care model with the purpose of improving practices related to the AVF.

2 Structured Nursing Care to the Arteriovenous Fistula

Vascular access, and particularly achieving a reliable and problem-free access, has always been a challenge for the scientific community throughout the evolution of dialysis. Vascular access plays a crucial role in hemodialysis outcomes, but it also represents a significant drain on financial resources and remains a leading cause of patient hospitalization. Medicare spends $2.8 billion on vascular access maintenance annually in the USA, corresponding to 12% of annual Medicare ESRD payments (Thamer et al. 2018).

Literature shows that the AVF is considered the best vascular access for haemodialysis. It has few problems and better patency when compared to other types of vascular access (graft or central venous catheter). The dialysis team (nephrologists and nephrologist nurses) and the patient need to carry out specific care in order to keep the AVF in the best conditions for haemodialysis treatment. Patients and all the elements of the dialysis team have their own requirements to contribute to access patency.

Nephrologist nurses can have a major contribution concerning prevention and detection of complications during the cannulation process, treatment and providing information on AVF care to patients (Sousa 2012). However, literature shows that nursing practices involved in the treatment (monitor preparation or patient connection to the monitor, among others) are carried out separately, failing to establish the integration of the different AVF features and to relate them to the patient's needs (Sousa et al. 2014; Pessoa et al. 2020). Such partitioning of nursing practice does not allow the identification of the nephrologist nurse's contribution as an important element of the dialysis team in the improvement of nephrological care provided to patients with ESRD (Sousa 2012), nor the development of sensitive indicators of nursing care related to vascular access. A model or structure of nursing care focused on vascular access, specifically the AVF, can be found in the literature.

In fact, Sousa (2012) proposed a structured care approach aimed at guiding and improving nursing practice with the arteriovenous access through specific nursing interventions. Sousa's structure enables the organization of care practices and the development of attention areas through implementation of practices that increase patency and minimize AVF thrombosis.

This structure has two areas of care: self-care (patient-oriented) and surveillance (nurse-oriented). Each area is made up of several related concepts complementing each other. Thus, it provides specific guidelines for care practice to patients with AVF (Fig. 1).

Self-Care Area

In the area of self-care, the patient must develop self-care behaviours to take care of his/her own AVF. The nurse plays an important role to promote the development of such behaviours through the information he/she provides the patient. In the course of the self-care training process, the nurse encourages the patient to use the potential to build up knowledge, skills and behaviours on AVF care (Sousa et al. 2021). Thus, learning self-care behaviours enables the patient to develop skills and abilities that can detect and avoid situations likely to cause AVF dysfunction (Sousa 2012).

The self-care area consists of four dimensions temporally defined according to the stages of CKD: anticipatory self-care in the creation of the AVF; self-care in 48 hours after creation of the AVF; self-care during AVF maturation and self-care with AVF in haemodialysis (Sousa 2012). The dimension term means a set of nursing care procedures to be provided to the patient with AVF in a given period in order to promote his/her self-care behaviours. The nurse can use a number of teaching strategies to train the patient for self-care.

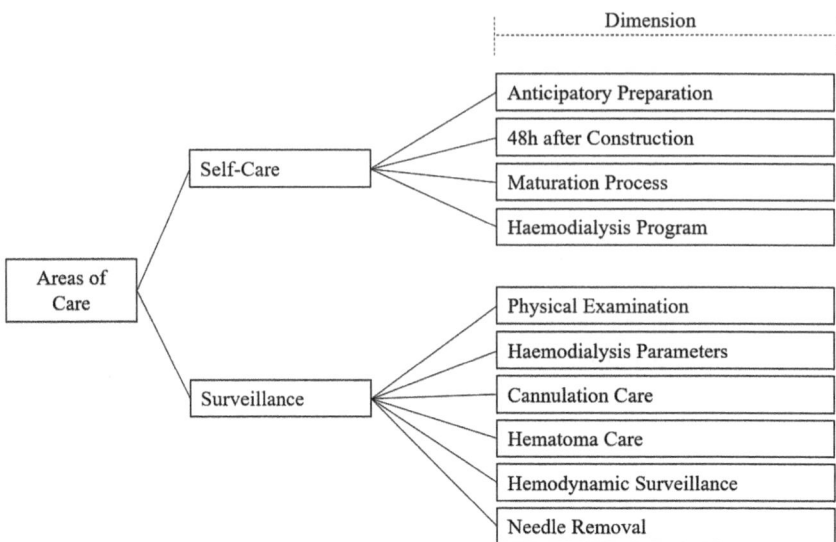

Fig. 1 Structure of nursing care focused on arteriovenous fistula (Sousa 2012)

The dimension of anticipatory self-care in the creation of the AVF corresponds to the period from the diagnosis of CKD to the creation of the AVF. The nurse's intervention should be targeted to enable patients develop their self-care behaviours seeking the preservation of the vascular network (Sousa 2012).

Several vascular access guidelines mention the importance of the patient carrying out self-care behaviours to preserve the network (Kukita et al. 2015; Ibeas et al. 2017; Lok et al. 2020). The quality of the vascular network (arterial and venous) can influence the process of AVF's creation and maturation. The vascular network of patients with CKD is subject to numerous external traumas, mainly cannulations; blood samples; intravenous medication; peripherally or centrally inserted venous catheters; and invasive exams (Sousa et al. 2018).

The dimension of self-care in the 48 hours after AVF creation corresponds to the time span of 48 hours after AVF creation. Patients must carry out their self-care behaviours in order to learn the skills required to prevent or early detect AVF thrombosis in this period.

During the maturation process, the nurse must promote patients' self-care behaviours in four specific areas of AVF care and his/her intervention should be directed to functionality; hypoperfusion complications; immediate care; functionality conservation. Concerning functionality, patients must be able to identify the thrill of the AVF and to enhance venous return (Sousa 2012). Patients should be informed and trained to identify signs and symptoms of distal hypoperfusion syndrome, mainly loss of sensitivity; cooling of the extremities or functional loss of the hand. These problems correspond to hypoperfusion complications.

The dimension of self-care with AVF in haemodialysis corresponds to the time span from the first cannulation to AVF thrombosis. The nurse's intervention should seek the maintenance of the vascular access in the best possible conditions (Sousa 2012). Literature shows that the state of the vascular access can influence treatment effectiveness.

The nurse must promote patients' self-care behaviours in five specific areas of AVF care in the context of haemodialysis: pre-cannulation care; intradialytic care; care in removing needles; hematoma care and interdialytic care. Concerning the first one, training patients is the goal so that care can decrease and avoid transmission of infection. Regarding the second, the nurse must train the patient to recognize the signs and symptoms of dialysis-induced hypotension and teach him/her to wear appropriate clothing. The third is about explaining the patient the importance of appropriate compression at the cannulation sites through dynamic pressure. The fourth concerns how the nurse trains the patient on home care with hematomas, particularly on ice or heparinoid ointment application. Interdialytic care is an essential part of the information to be provided to the patient on self-care behaviours designed both to prevent complications and to manage signs and symptoms (Sousa 2012).

A number of studies show that the frequency of self-care behaviours with AVF is lower than expected (Pessoa and Linhares 2015; Sousa et al. 2017, 2020, 2021, 2022). In fact, a very large proportion of patients, such as up to nearly 98%, may skip those behaviours (Pessoa and Linhares 2015). This is a real problem that must be dealt with by the nephrologist nurse. Since the patient is the person who suffers in case of problems with the AVF, he/she should develop self-care behaviours to take care of it properly.

These four dimensions can enable the development of an educational approach in order to promote self-care in ESRD patients with AVF, through the development of nursing therapies in a training, guiding, describing and explaining framework (Sousa 2012).

Surveillance Area

In the surveillance area, the nephrologist nurse must have an integrative approach through the different dimensions, especially concerning those aspects related to preparation, creation and maintenance of the AVF (Fig. 2). Care with the AVF should start prior to its creation and continue during its creation, maturation and later in its use in haemodialysis.

Literature shows nurses' contribution in the pre- and post-creation stage and when complications associated with the AVF occur, being considered a central and extremely important pillar to maintaining the quality of access.

This area is made up of six dimensions: physical examination; haemodialysis parameters; cannulation care; haematoma care; haemodynamic surveillance and care in needle removal (Sousa 2012). In each dimension, depending on its own specificity, nursing interventions were associated with the objective of developing cognitive competence and skills that enable nurses to assess the vascular access.

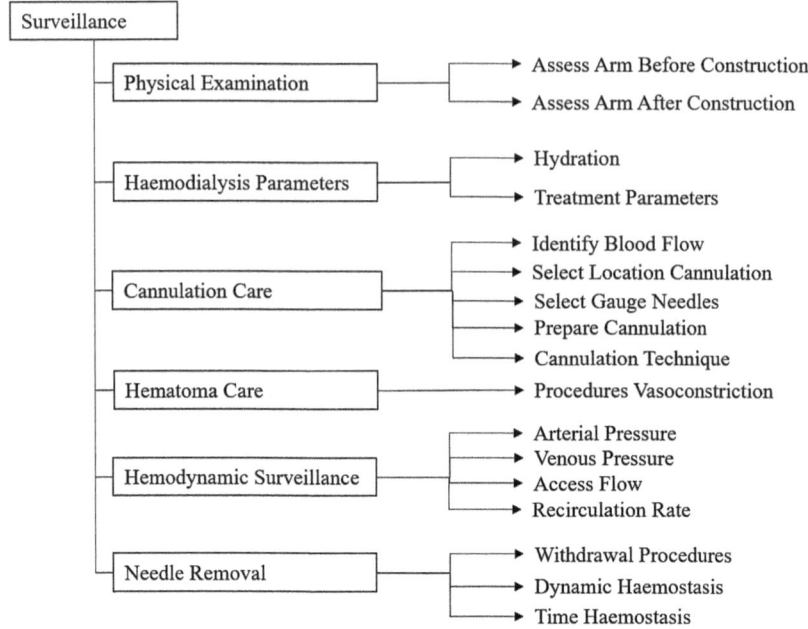

Fig. 2 Area of care: surveillance (Sousa 2012)

Concerning the first dimension, physical examination, the nurse must assess the limb of the access or future access seeking to find objective and subjective information to prevent complications related to the vascular access. Physical examination consists of a set of procedures to be carried out on the patient by observation, palpation and auscultation. Physical examination should be performed prior to access making in order to identify which upper limb may provide better conditions for making the AVF (Sousa 2012). Furthermore, physical examination after AVF creation seeks to detect complications or situations that may compromise the development and maintenance of the AVF.

In the dimension of haemodialysis parameters, the nurse is expected to develop care practice to prevent, detect and implement interventions seeking to decrease dialysis-induced hypotension. In this dimension, it is also important to consider and analyse the patient's fluid-status parameters and change the dialysis strategy (Sousa 2012).

Concerning cannulation care, the nurse has a major contribution to identify the best cannulation sites. Fistula cannulation should not be restricted to the cannulation technique because other aspects are extremely important in this process, namely identification of blood flow; selection of appropriate cannulation sites; needle selection; cannulation site preparation and cannulation technique (Sousa 2012; Pinto et al. 2022). During this process, the nurse must use ultrasound to analyse the vein morphology (depth, diameter, sites with reduced diameter) and to identify the segment to be punctured. Nurses ought to interrelate the different aspects of this dimension with the aim of developing strategies to save the patient's vascular network and to improve the permeability of the vascular access.

In the dimension of haematoma care, nurses must carry out care practices seeking to reduce the impact of haematomas or infiltrations. A set of nursing interventions are available in order to minimize the effects of hematomas/infiltrations and to enable the success of the vascular access during puncture (Sousa 2012).

Regarding haemodynamic surveillance, analysing and monitoring the AVF pressure profile from effective interpretation of data displayed by the haemodialysis monitor are required in order to detect access dysfunction. Monitoring arterial and venous pressures, assessing blood flow (by direct and indirect methods), assessing the relationship between intra-access pressure and mean arterial pressure (IAP/MAP), and determining the recirculation rate are essential parameters for detecting AVF dysfunction (Sousa 2012).

Nurses must articulate these aspects of surveillance and monitoring in order to develop and implement programmes seeking the detection of problems with the AVF.

The dimension of care of needle removal is related to the importance of careful needle removal, because it is as important as their insertion, in order to prevent post-dialysis trauma and haematomas. This dimension describes the shape and order of needle removal and the performance of appropriate dynamic haemostasis (performed by the nurse or the patient) (Sousa 2012). Dynamic haemostasis should be carried out in a gentle way in order to prevent blood loss and the full obstruction of blood flow in the vascular access. Static haemostasis with clamps or other objects that cause continuous and constant pressure on the AVF should be avoided (Sousa 2012).

3 Practical Implications

Nurses are health professionals who are in direct contact with the vascular access and handle the AVF. The existence of a structured care with areas of attention can promote the development of cognitive competence and the acquisition of skills, enabling nurses to identify and diagnose changes in the AVF performance. Such structured care can also show the contribution of nurses to the efficiency of health care in the area of nephrology.

References

Bello A, Okpechi I, Osman M, Cho Y, Htay H, Jha V, Johnson D (2022) Epidemiology of haemodialysis outcomes. Nat Rev Nephrol 18(6):378–395

Brescia M, Cimino J, Appel K, Hurwich B (1966) Chronic hemodialysis using venepuncture and a surgically created arteriovenous fistula. N Engl J Med 275(20):1089–1092

Clementi A, Coppolino G, Provenzano M, Granata A, Battaglia G (2021) The holistic vision of the patient with chronic kidney disease in an universalistic health care system. Ther Apher Dial 25(2):136–144. https://doi.org/10.1111/1744-9987.13556

Coelho A, Sá H, Diniz J, Dussault G (2014) The integrated management for renal replacement therapy in Portugal. Hemodial Int 18(1):175–184

Dagher F, Gelber R, Ramos E, Sadler J (1976) The use of basilic vein and brachial artery as an A-V fistula for long term hemodialysis. J Surg Res 20(4):373–376

Fukasawa M (2019) Current status of vascular access in Japan—from Dialysis Access Symposium 2017. J Vasc Access 20(1_suppl):38–44

Ibeas J, Roca-Tey R, Vallespín J, Moreno T, Moñux G, Martí-Monrós A et al (2017) Spanish clinical guidelines on vascular access for haemodialysis. Nefrologia 37(Suppl 1):1–191

Jager K, Kovesdy C, Langham R, Rosenberg M, Jha V, Zoccali C (2019) A single number for advocacy and communication-worldwide more than 850 million individuals have kidney diseases. Kidney Int 96:1048–1050

Kukita K, Ohira S, Amano I, Naito H, Azuma N, Ikeda K et al (2015) 2011 update Japanese Society for Dialysis Therapy Guidelines of Vascular Access Construction and Repair for Chronic Hemodialysis. Ther Apher Dial 19(Suppl 1):1–39

Lok C, Huber T, Lee T, Shenoy S, Yevzlin A, Abreo K et al (2020) KDOQI clinical practice guideline for vascular access: 2019 update. Am J Kidney Dis 75(4 Suppl 2):S1–S164

Pessoa N, Linhares F (2015) Hemodialysis patients with arteriovenous fistula: knowledge, attitude and practice. Esc Anna Nery 19(1):73–79

Pessoa N, Lima L, Santos G, Frazão C, Sousa C, Ramos V (2020) Self-care actions for the maintenance of the arteriovenous fistula: an integrative review. Int J Nurs Sc 7(3):369–377

Pinto R, Sousa C, Salgueiro A, Fernandes I (2022) Arteriovenous fistula cannulation in hemodialysis: a vascular access clinical practice guidelines narrative review. J Vasc Access 23(5):825–831

Sato T, Sakurai H, Okubo K, Kusuta R, Onogi T, Tsuboi M (2019) Current state of dialysis treatment and vascular access management in Japan. J Vasc Access 20(1_suppl):10–14

Sousa C (2012) Caring for the person arteriovenous fistula: model for continuous improvement. Rev Port Sau Pub 30(1):11–17

Sousa C, Apóstolo J, Figueiredo M, Martins M, Dias V (2014) Interventions to promote self-care of people with arteriovenous fistula. J Clin Nurs 23(13-14):1796–1802

Sousa C, Marujo P, Teles P, Lira M, Novais M (2017) Self-care on hemodialysis: behaviors with the arteriovenous fistula. Ther Apher Dial 21(2):195–199

Sousa C, Ligeiro I, Teles P, Paixão L, Dias V, Cristovão A (2018) Self-care in preserving the vascular network: old problem, new challenge for the medical staff. Ther Apher Dial 22(4):332–336

Sousa C, Marujo P, Teles P, Lira M, Dias V, Novais M (2020) Self-care behavior profiles with arteriovenous fistula in hemodialysis patients. Clin Nurs Res 29(6):363–367

Sousa C, Paquete A, Teles P, Pinto C, Dias V, Ribeiro O et al (2021) Investigating the effect of a structured intervention on the development of self-care behaviors with arteriovenous fistula in hemodialysis patients. Clin Nurs Res 30(6):866–874

Sousa C, Teles P, Paquete A, Dias V, Manzini C, Nicole A et al (2022) Effects of demographic and clinical character on differences in self-care behavior levels with arteriovenous fistula by hemodialysis patients: an ordinal logistic regression approach. Ther Apher Dial 26(5):992–998

Thamer M, Lee T, Wasse H, Glickman M, Qian J, Gottlieb D et al (2018) Medicare costs associated with arteriovenous fistulas among US hemodialysis patients. Am J Kidney Dis 72(1):10–18

Thurlow J, Joshi M, Yan G, Norris K, Agodoa L, Yuan C, Nee R (2021) Global epidemiology of end-stage kidney disease and disparities in kidney replacement therapy. Am J Nephrol 52(2):98–107

Creation of an Arteriovenous Fistula

Clemente Neves Sousa, Nurten Ozen, and António Norton de Matos

The process of creating a vascular access is complex and several issues must be considered in order to increase the number of arteriovenous fistulas (AVF) such as assessing the patient (age, sex, dominant arm, comorbidity, and kidney-disease etiology), the risk of vascular-access complications (risk of central stenosis, distal hypoperfusion, and risk of thrombosis/bleeding), and the vascular network (arterial and venous network).

The existence of a proper vascular network is crucial for a successful access. The patient must have an arterial and venous network compatible with the creation of an AVF. Knowing which vascular network is used in the AVF and particularly the anatomy of the arterial and venous network has a major importance.

1 Arterial Network

The arterial system of the upper limb is made up of a series of arteries that supply blood to the arm, forearm, hand, and fingers. The subclavian artery passes over the first rib and becomes the axillary artery. Furthermore, the axillary artery is called the brachial

C. N. Sousa (✉)
Nursing School of University of Portto, Porto, Portugal
e-mail: clementesousa@esenf.pt

RISE – Health, University of Porto, Porto, Portugal

N. Ozen
Faculty of Nursing, Department of Internal Medicine Nursing, Istanbul University, Istanbul, Turkey
e-mail: nurten.ozen@istanbul.edu.tr

A. Norton de Matos
Grupo de Estudos Vasculares (Vascular Access Center), Porto, Portugal

© The Author(s), under exclusive license to Springer Nature Switzerland AG 2025
N. Ozen et al. (eds.), *Arteriovenous Fistula Management*,
https://doi.org/10.1007/978-3-032-04771-7_2

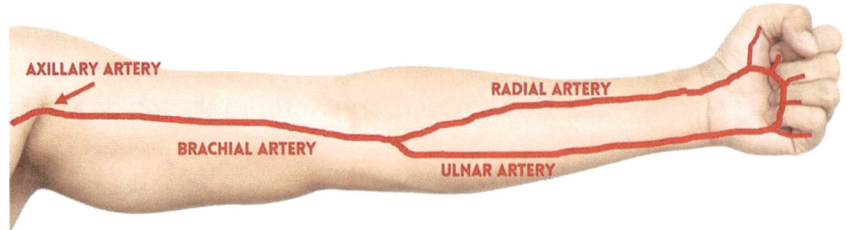

Fig. 1 Arterial network (image was adapted, with type of word: Lovelo, N.:º 14)

artery when it reaches the arm. The brachial artery runs down the arm and bifurcates into two smaller arteries, the radial artery and the ulnar artery, approximately 2 cm below the elbow. The radial and ulnar arteries communicate with each other forming the palmar arch in the palm of the hand (Fig. 1).

2 Venous Network

The venous system is constituted by the superficial venous system and the deep venous system. At the level of the forearm, the superficial venous system is formed by the cephalic vein that begins at the wrist and can run along the outer surface of the forearm or the inner face. When the cephalic vein of the forearm is more external, it normally communicates directly with the cephalic vein of the arm approximately 2 cm above the elbow. The cephalic vein of the forearm can be displaced by the internal surface, giving rise to the median vein of the forearm, which, in turn, can bifurcate through the median cephalic vein and the median basilic vein at the level of the elbow. Anatomical variations of the forearm veins are common in the forearm, so the venous network must receive special attention. Anatomical variations of the cephalic vein have been classified into three most frequent types based on the anatomical location of the forearm of the cephalic vein (Fig. 2).

In type A variation, the cephalic vein in the middle third drains into the median vein in the forearm, then into the median basilic vein and subsequently into the basilic vein. In type B variation, the cephalic vein in the transition from the middle to the upper third of the forearm bifurcates through the cephalic vein (subsequently through the cephalic vein of the arm) and through the median basilic vein (subsequently through the basilic vein). In type C variation, the cephalic vein is located on the outer surface of the forearm and continues into the upper arm. The median vein of the forearm is located on the inner surface, communicating with the median basilic and median cephalic vein, which subsequently communicates with the cephalic vein of the arm.

The cephalic vein runs down the central aspect of the arm and merges with the subclavian vein. The area where the cephalic vein meets the subclavian vein is called

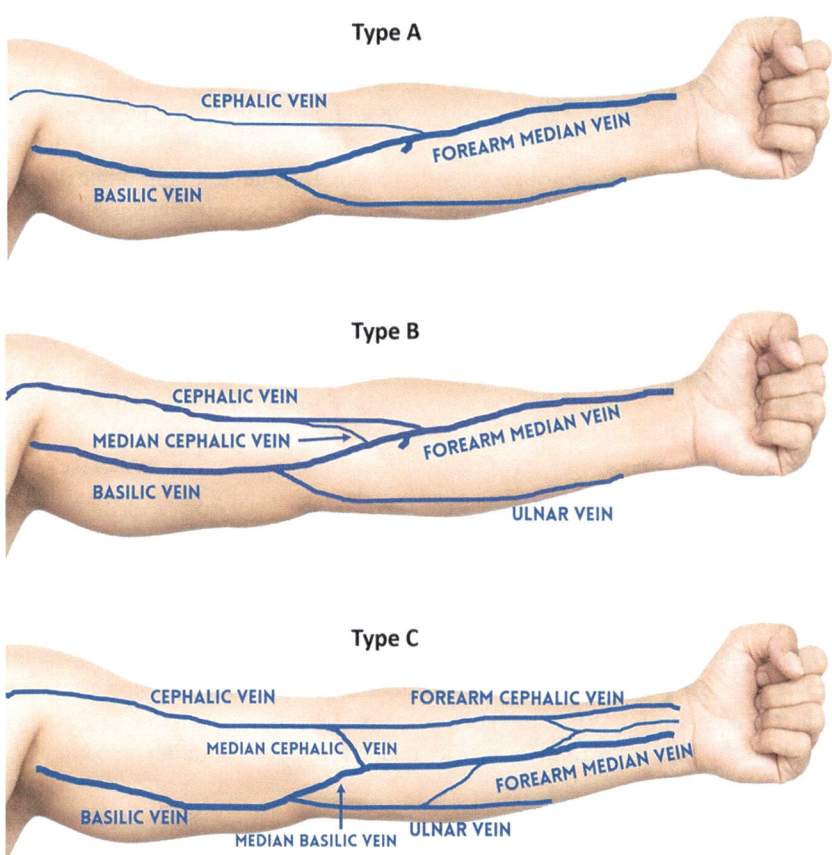

Fig. 2 Three most frequent types of the cephalic vein forearm (image was adapted, with type of word: Lovelo, N:° 14)

the cephalic arch. The ulnar or basilic vein begins at the wrist and runs along the posterior surface of the forearm. In the elbow area, approximately 2 cm above the elbow, the ulnar vein merges with the basilic vein of the arm, which in turn merges with the axillary vein at the level of the armpit.

Venous drainage is also provided by the deep venous system. Such drainage is usually carried out by veins with the same name as the arteries. Normally, two radial veins and two ulnar veins accompany the respective arteries, communicating with the superficial veins through several tributary veins. The radial and ulnar veins will unite to form the perforating or deep vein of the forearm at the arm level. The deep vein is called the brachial vein and drains into the axillary vein.

3 Creation of Arteriovenous Fistula

AVF's classical creation technique was described by Brescia-Cimino in 1966 and it has evolved to this day. There are different techniques to create the anastomosis of the artery (always adopting the sequence of artery to vein). Historically, the first anastomosis was created through the side-to-side technique. Later, other types of anastomosis techniques were developed such as the end-to-end technique, end-to-side technique, and side-to-end technique (Konner 2005). The anastomosis technique most commonly used today in distal AVF is the side-to-end anastomosis.

The four anastomosis techniques have advantages and disadvantages. The side-to-side anastomosis is technically simple to perform and allows a good flow. The downside is that it can cause venous hypertension syndrome with functional changes in the hand. The end-to-end anastomosis has the advantage of directing the flow only to the vein, avoiding loss of flow to the distal part. However, this technique is more demanding for the vascular surgeon and may predispose to distal hypoperfusion and ischemia, especially in diabetic and elderly patients. The side-to-end anastomosis has become the technique preferred by vascular surgeons to create an AVF. It is more suited when the vein is not so close to the artery (without creating an acute angle) facilitating the creation of the fistula. In this type of anastomosis, thrombosis generally occurs, when it does, in the venous segment only, not compromising the artery. However, this anastomosis technique may have some problems, with a higher failure rate or maturation problems.

The AVF can be created at the wrist, forearm, antecubital fossa, upper arm, and thigh. Creation of the AVF at the wrist is the best location, due to the lower rate of complications but it may raise difficulties concerning the maturation process.

4 Types of Arteriovenous Fistula

The radial artery and cephalic vein of the forearm are usually selected for creation of an AVF in the forearm. However, other veins (ulnar vein and forearm median vein) and the ulnar artery can be used in the creation. It is important during the selection process to identify the vascular network suitable for creation of an AVF by using ultrasound.

Distal Fistulas

Distal fistulas are the best solution and the first option for the arteriovenous access for hemodialysis patients (Ibeas et al. 2017; Kukita et al. 2015; Lok et al. 2020). One of the problems of this type of fistula is the greater primary failure and inappropriate maturation to start the puncture (Ibeas et al. 2017). Distal fistulas can be created in the snuffbox, wrist, and forearm.

Snuffbox Arteriovenous Fistula

Vascular access guidelines recommend making the AVF as distal as possible when feasible. The most distal AVF of the forearm is in the snuffbox, located on the volar surface of the hand. This type of AVF was described in 1969 by Rassat et al. (1969) and is characterized by creation of a side-to-end anastomosis between the radial artery and the cephalic vein, which are very close, making it the ideal place to create such an AVF. However, this type of AVF is not commonly created. Inappropriate vascular network or anatomical changes, patient preference, choice of vascular surgeon, or unfamiliarity with the procedure are variables that can make it difficult to create a snuffbox AVF.

Several studies have shown that the snuffbox AVF has the same results as the fistula at the wrist, being a good option when the patient has a proper vascular network to create the fistula in this location (Heindel et al. 2021; Siracuse et al. 2019). The creation of the snuffbox AVF can vary between 4% and 17.6%, depending on the series (Siracuse et al. 2019; Heindel et al. 2021). This type of fistula can be difficult to create in patients with the following characteristics: old age, problems related to the vein (elasticity, synechia, continuity with forearm veins, and diameter) and artery (calcification and diameter) (Idrees et al. 2020; Mokhtari et al. 2022). However, the vascular access guidelines suggest the creation of the autogenous access should be as distal as possible in order to increase the length of the draining vein. This strategy also increases and preserves the options for future access.

Literature shows the feasibility and efficiency of creating a snuffbox AVF. A systematic review, which included 1503 snuffbox fistulas from 1982 to 2015, showed patency rates ranging from 61% to 87% at 1-year follow-up and decreasing to 36.3%–87% at longer follow-up (Idrees et al. 2020). Another study, analyzing 55 sunffbox AVFs, found a secondary patency at 1 year equal to 92.3% (95% CI, 85.3%–99.9%) (Heindel et al. 2021). The clinical maturation rate at 1 year was 83.7% ($n=55$; 95% CI, 66.8%–91.9%) and the functional maturation rate at 1 year was 85.6% ($n=40$; 95% CI, 63.3%–94.4% (Heindel et al. 2021).

The maturation process can be a problem for a sunffbox AVF. However, in a study with 47 patients (39 wrist and 8 snuffbox AVFs), the frequency of primary maturation failure was the same, with no significant differences (47.2% of wrist and 50% snuffbox fistulas) (Mokhtari et al. 2022). The demographic characteristic and comorbidities of the patients can influence the maturation of the sunffbox AVF.

Radiocephalic Arteriovenous Fistula

Literature shows that the radiocephalic AVF is considered the best vascular access for hemodialysis treatment since it has few complications and high patency when its maturation process is smooth. Such an AVF was first created on February 19, 1965 by surgeon Dr. Appell, through a side-to-side anastomosis between the radial artery and the cephalic vein (Konner 2005). The results of this technique were impressive, with no cases of primary failure, complications, or thrombosis. In 1966, Brescia et al.

(1966) published the article *"Chronic hemodialysis using venipuncture and surgically created arteriovenous fistula"* after 16 months of use of fistulas in hemodialysis patients.

The radiocephalic AVF is created as far down the arm as possible, usually at the wrist. However, in older patients or those with venous network diameter problems, the AVF can be created approximately 5 cm above the wrist, when the dorsal vein of the hand converges with the cephalic vein of the forearm. The anastomosis between the radial artery and the cephalic vein described by Brescia et al. was side-to-side. Such type of anastomosis can promote the venous-hypertension syndrome at the level of the hand. Currently, in this type of AVF, anastomosis is performed in the side-to-end to avoid hand problems.

The disadvantage of the radiocephalic AVF is non-maturation, characterized by inappropriate dimensions of the draining vein or insufficient blood flow. The ratio of non-maturation cases of such an AVF relative to the arm AVF is only 24% (Voorzaat et al. 2018). This situation can delay the removal of the central venous catheter, compromise the start of dialysis, or favor access thrombosis. However, a radiocephalic AVF can be created more proximally to the hand, reducing the risk of steal syndrome, hemodialysis-access-induced distal ischemia (HAIDI) or high-flow access (Ibeas et al. 2017).

Ulnarbasilic Arteriovenous Fistula

The ulnarbasilic fistula was first reported by Hanson et al. (1967). This type of fistula is uncommon due to the reduced diameter of the ulnar artery or the small caliber of the ulnar vein or basilic vein of the forearm. The creation of the ulnarbasilic fistula consists of the connection through a side-to-end anastomosis between the ulnar artery and the ulnar vein or basilic vein of the forearm. The primary patency of this type of fistulas can average between 70.9% and 73.8% in the first 12 months (Salgado et al. 2004; Sharma et al. 2021), and it may achieve 57.3% after 5 years without any procedure to maintain survival of the fistula (Salgado et al. 2004).

Such a fistula can be an alternative to the proximal access but it must be specifically selected for patients with an appropriate vascular network (arterial and venous).

Radiobasilic Arteriovenous Fistula (Transposition)

In some situations, the diameter of the ulnar/basilic vein is good enough for a fistula, but the ulnar artery is not compatible with the access. In 1980, Lindstert and Lindergard (1980) described a new technique for transposing the basilic vein of the forearm with six incisions, creating a radial-basilic fistula in the forearm. This fistula consists of the connection through a side-to-end anastomosis between the radial artery and the ulnar/basilic vein which is moved to the inner side of the forearm. Only a few studies on this technique are available, but maturation time varies between 45.2 ± 10.7 days (mean $\pm$ standard deviation) and 49.85 ± 5.66 days, patency is 12.67 ± 5.83 months, and primary assisted patency is 21.33 ± 4.61 months, with patency ranging between 77% and 90.5% (Uzun et al. 2019; Khan et al. 2023). This type of fistula favors access cannulation by the nurse.

Proximal Fistulas

Proximal fistulas, in the antecubital fossa, are the second option after distal fistulas (Ibeas et al. 2017). Antecubital fossa fistulas are usually made with larger diameter vessels, which cause greater blood flow and less maturation problems. Upper arm fistulas have a better maturation process than forearm fistulas (55% and 16% after 6 weeks, respectively) (Robbin et al. 2016). This flow causes less problems with primary failure but worsens problems with drainage, mainly in the cephalic arch, steal syndrome, HAIDI, and high flow access (Ibeas et al. 2017; Kukita et al. 2015; Lok et al. 2020; Teixeira et al. 2017).

Brachiocephalic Arteriovenous Fistula

The brachiocephalic arteriovenous fistula is the first choice for creating a fistula in the upper arm. The construction of this type of fistula depends on the anatomy and configuration of the venous network. Such an access can be created into the cephalic vein or into the median cephalic vein with anastomosis of the brachial artery, through a side-to-end anastomosis. However, depending on the patient's venous network, it may be possible to construct a fistula close to the perforating vein. This fistula usually arterializes the cephalic and basilic veins and became known as Gracz fistula.

A study with 2359 patients on hemodialysis compared primary patency in patients with brachiocephalic (1389 patients) and with radiocephalic (970 patients) arteriovenous fistulas after 1 year (Plauche et al. 2023). Primary patency was 45% vs. 41.3% respectively ($p=0.88$), assisted primary patency was 86.7% versus 86.9% ($p=0.64$), the absence of reintervention was 51.1% versus 46.3% ($p=0.44$), and survival was 81.3% versus 84.9% ($p=0.02$) (Plauche et al. 2023).

Brachiobasilic Arteriovenous Fistula (Transposition)

The basilic vein is a good choice for fistula creation because it is a deep vein, it is protected from the subcutaneous tissue, and usually it is not used for cannulation. Dagher first described the brachiobasilic arteriovenous fistula and its transposition in 1976 (Dagher et al. 1976). However, superficialization or transposition of the basilic vein is required after making a brachiobasilic fistula. Superficialization means placing the basilic vein closer to the skin, i.e., more superficially, while transposition consists of displacing and superficializing the basilic vein to the external face of the arm. Transposition can be done with only three small incisions of about 1 cm each in order to dissect and transpose the vein (Rego et al. 2018). Basilic transposition is generally performed in two steps, the first to create the fistula and the second to carry out the superficialization or transposition.

The primary patency rate at 12 months of basilic vein transposition was 50.8%, and the assisted primary and secondary patency rates at 12 months were 82.4% and 84.0%, respectively (Rego et al. 2018). Secondary patency of the transposed basilic vein at 1, 2, and 3 years may vary from 54% to 90%, 38% to 82%, and 43% to 57%, respectively, depending on the studies (Rego et al. 2018).

Brachiobrachial Arteriovenous Fistula (Transposition)

The absence of superficial veins or when the vein diameter is not suitable for a fistula may require the creation of a fistula in the deep venous system. For such patients, the brachial vein may be a good option for an autologous vascular access. The creation of a brachiobrachial arteriovenous fistula will only be possible if the patient has more than one brachial vein. Koontz and Helling (1983) first described the brachiobrachial arteriovenous fistula and its transposition. In 2017, Norton de Matos et al. presented a new technique with a short skip incisions (Norton de Matos et al. 2017). The surgery required by such a fistula has to be carried out in two stages, the first to create the fistula and the second to perform brachial transposition.

The maturation time between the first and the second stages of surgery is long, with an average time of 99.4 days (range: 47–164 days) (Sha et al. 2016). After transposition, the average time to cannulation is 50.8 days (range: 17–103 days) (Sha et al. 2016). This type of vascular access may take 3–6 months for cannulation to start. Primary patency rate at 12 months ranged between 24% and 77% in a study of 380 brachiobrachial arteriovenous fistulas (Norton de Matos et al. 2017). Secondary patency is similar to that of brachiobasilic arteriovenous fistula transposition (Kim et al. 2020).

5 Maturation Process of Arteriovenous Fistula

The maturation process depends on three variables that must work well with each other: cardiac output, arterial inflow, and venous outflow (Dinwiddie 2002). The articulation of these variables allows an appropriate arterial pressure in the peripheral arterial system, so that the blood flow can pass to the venous system with proper pressure in order to develop the vein.

The arterial system is considered to have high resistance and high pressure, while the venous system has lower resistance and pressure. When the fistula is created, blood from the arterial system (high pressure) will run into the venous system which has less resistance. The increase in blood pressure in the venous system (it receives a high-pressure flow) leads to a rise in the venous diameter and to thickening of the venous wall (Ahmad 2000). Usually, loss of perfusion in other vascular areas (e.g., hand) is avoided by compensatory mechanisms with a reflex raise in cardiac output, increasing the injection volume and cardiac contractility without increasing the pulse (Arroyo-Bielsa et al. 2005). This mechanism enables keeping a stable blood pressure and increasing the blood flow to the fistula.

The fistula flow increases significantly in the artery and anastomosis and decreases in intensity along the draining vein. The average blood flow in the radial artery is less than 25 ml/min, while in the brachial artery it is 50 ml/min at rest (Joannides et al. 1997; Lomonte et al. 2005). However, mean artery blood flow will be increased by less than 10–20 times, to a minimum of 500 ml/min. This change in the vascular structure is explained by Poiseuille's Law, which determines that the flow (Q) is proportional to the product of the pressure gradient (ΔP) and the radial vein (r) raised to the fourth, divided by the progression of the blood (η) ($Q \propto \Delta P \times r^4/\eta$) (Dixon 2006).

In order to accommodate the increased blood flow from the fistula, the vein will undergo a process of dilation and wall thickening. Vein dilation can occur quickly, after creating the fistula, and last for several weeks. A number of studies show that the increase in vein diameter in a fistula can range from an interval between 56% and 86% on the first day after fistula creation, to an interval between 123% and 179% after 12 weeks (Wong et al. 1996; Corpataux et al. 2002). The fistula's blood flow increases rapidly right after construction of the artery–vein anastomosis, followed immediately by a progressive increase in flow, reaching its maximum within 4–12 weeks (Wong et al. 1996; Lomonte et al. 2005). Even though the blood flow rate changes, the fistula reaches 40%–60% of its maximum flow on the first day after anastomosis (Wong et al. 1996; Lomonte et al. 2005). The maximum flow can be reached in 4 weeks in a forearm fistula (Asif et al. 2006).

Time of the maturation process is not clearly defined in the literature, but there exists a correlation between flow, vein diameter, and depth. Several authors consider different aspects to identify the appropriate maturation of the fistula. According to Dember et al. (2005), a fistula was considered mature if it achieved a blood flow of at least 300 ml/min during eight or more sessions, that is, 30 days. Dixon (2006) defined fistula maturation as achieving sufficient blood flow to sustain a haemodialysis session (at least 350–400 ml/min), along with a vein diameter large enough to allow the insertion of two needles, enabling three to five hours of effective treatment. Other authors claim it is important to acknowledge the risk of bleeding when cannulation occurs (Rayner et al. 2003), the risk of infiltration, an appropriate access flow rate ≥ 500 ml/min (Patel et al. 2003) or when the vein is superficial enough to identify sites for safe cannulation (Lok et al. 2020). Some of these subjectively assessed aspects may make it difficult to identify an appropriate maturation. KDOQI Vascular Access Guidelines (2006) (Vascular Access 2006) defined fistula maturation according to the 6s rule (at least 6 mm in diameter, less than 6 mm in depth, blood flow greater than 600 ml/min, and assessment after 6 weeks of creation). This is one of the most used definitions of appropriate fistula maturation in the literature.

Clearly, there is no consensus on the definition of proper AVF maturation. However, all authors show the importance of assessing such an access through physical examination and ultrasound. Several vascular access guidelines recommend the use of ultrasound to identify appropriate maturation and problems that may compromise it (Lok et al. 2020; Ibeas et al. 2017; Schmidli et al. 2018).

6 Practical Implications

The patient must have a compatible arterial and venous network to create an arteriovenous fistula. The arterial network must provide an appropriate flow without compromising the distal circulation after AVF creation. The venous network must not present outflow problems. Such variables and the cardiac flow can influence the process of patency and maturation of the AVF. Likewise, personal characteristics (sex or obesity) and comorbidities (diabetes or peripherical arterial disease) can influence access maturation.

References

Ahmad S (2000). Manual of clinical dialysis. Science Press Ltd, Londres
Arroyo-Bielsa A, Gil-Sales J, Gesto-Castromil R (2005) Accesos vasculares para hemodiálisis: complicaciones hiperaflujo o flujo excesivo. Angiologia 57(Suppl 2):S109–S116
Asif A, Roy-Chaudhury P, Beathard G (2006) Early arteriovenous fistula failure: logical proposal for when and how to intervene. Clin J Am Soc Nephrol 1(2):332–339
Brescia M, Cimino J, Appel K, Hurwich B (1966) Chronic hemodialysis using venepuncture and a surgically created arteriovenous fistula. N Engl J Med 275(20):1089–1092
Corpataux J, Haesler E, Silacci P, Ris H, Hayoz D (2002) Low-pressure environment and remodelling of the forearm vein in Brescia-Cimino haemodialysis access. Nephrol Dial Transplant 17(6):1057–1062
Dagher F, Gelber R, Ramos E, Sadler J (1976) The use of basilic vein and brachial artery as an A-V fistula for long term hemodialysis. J Surg Res 20(4):373–376
Dember L, Kaufman J, Beck G, Dixon B, Gassman J, Greene T et al (2005) Design of the Dialysis Access Consortium (DAC) clopidogrel prevention of early AV fistula thrombosis trial. Clin Trials 2(5):413–422
Dinwiddie L (2002) Interventions to promote fistula maturation. Nephrol Nurs J 29(4):377–402
Dixon B (2006) Why don't fistulas mature?. Kidney Int 70(8):1413–1422
Hanson J, Carmody M, Keogh B, O'Dwyer W (1967) Access to circulation by permanent arteriovenous fistula in regular dialysis treatment. Br Med J 4(5579):586–589
Heindel PD, Sharma G, Belkin M, Ozaki C, Hentschel D (2021) Contemporary outcomes of a "snuffbox first" hemodialysis access approach in the United States. J Vasc Surg 74(3):947–956
Ibeas J, Roca-Tey R, Vallespín J, Moreno T, Moñux G, Martí-Monrós A et al (2017) Spanish clinical guidelines on vascular access for haemodialysis. Nefrologia 37(Suppl 1):1–191
Idrees M, Suthananthan A, Pathmarajah T, Sieunarine K (2020) Snuffbox fistula – a first-line approach to haemodialysis: a review. J Vasc Access 21(5):554–563
Joannides R, Bakkali E, Le Roy F, Rivault O, Godin M, Moore N et al (1997) Altered flow-dependent vasodilatation of conduit arteries in maintenance haemodialysis. Nephrol Dial Transplant 12(12):2623–2628
Khan U, Kareem T, Uneeb M, Ehsan O, Wyne H (2023) Forearm basilic vein transposition: a single-centre experience. Cureus 15(6):e40129. https://doi.org/10.7759/cureus.40129
Kim M, Min S, Ahn S, Kim H, Choi C, Mo H et al (2020) Modified brachio-basilic/brachial arteriovenous fistula creation with short-segment elevation preserving the axilla. Ann Vasc Surg 67:448.e1–448.e10
Konner K (2005) History of vascular access for haemodialysis. Nephrol Dial Transplant 20(12):2629–2635
Koontz PJ, Helling T (1983) Subcutaneous brachial vein arteriovenous fistula for chronic hemodialysis. World J Surg 7(5):672–674
Kukita K, Ohira S, Amano I, Naito H, Azuma N, Ikeda K et al (2015) 2011 update Japanese Society for Dialysis Therapy Guidelines of Vascular Access Construction and Repair for Chronic Hemodialysis. Ther Apher Dial 19(Suppl 1):1–39
Lindstedt E, Lindergård B (1980) Transposition of the basilic vein in the forearm for the construction of haemodialysis arteriovenous fistula. Scand J Urol Nephrol 14(2):207–209
Lok C, Huber T, Lee T, Shenoy S, Yevzlin A, Abreo K et al (2020) KDOQI clinical practice guideline for vascular access: 2019 update. Am J Kidney Dis 75(4 Suppl 2):S1–S164
Lomonte C, Casucci F, Antonelli M, Giammaria B, Losurdo N, Marchio G et al (2005) Is there a place for duplex screening of the brachial artery in the maturation of arteriovenous fistulas? Semin Dial 18(3):243–246
Mokhtari S, Besancenot A, Beaumont M, Leroux F, Rinckenbach S, Salomon Du Mont L (2022) Snuff-box versus wrist radiocephalic arteriovenous fistulas for hemodialysis: maturation tend and its affecting factors. Ann Vasc Surg 87:495–501. https://doi.org/10.1016/j.avsg.2022.05.032

Norton de Matos A, Sousa C, Almeida P, Queirós J, Rego D, Teixeira G et al (2017) Brachio-brachial arteriovenous fistula superficialization with short skip incisions. Ann Vasc Surg 41(4):311–313

Patel S, Hughes J, Mills J (2003) Failure of arteriovenous fistula maturation: an unintended consequence of exceeding dialysis outcome quality Initiative guidelines for hemodialysis access. J Vasc Surg 38(3):439–445

Plauche L, Farber A, King E, Levin S, Cheng T, Rybin D et al (2023) Brachiocephalic and radiocephalic arteriovenous fistulas in patients with tunneled dialysis catheters have similar outcomes. Ann Vasc Surg 12(23):S0890–S5096. https://doi.org/10.1016/j.avsg.2023.04.032

Rassat J, Moskovtchenko, Perrin J, Traeger J (1969) Artero-venous fistula in the anatomical snuff-box. J Urol Nephrol (Paris) 75(12 Suppl 12):482

Rayner H, Pisoni R, Gillespie B, Goodkin D, Akiba T, Akizawa T et al (2003) Creation, cannulation and survival of arteriovenous fistulae: data from the Dialysis Outcomes and Practice Patterns Study. Kidney Int 63(1):323–330

Rego D, Nogueira C, Matos A, Almeida P, Queirós J, Silva F et al (2018) Two-stage basilic vein transposition: second stage results. Ther Apher Dial 22(1):73–78

Robbin ML, Greene T, Cheung A, Allon M, Berceli SA, Kaufman JS (2016) Arteriovenous fistula development in the first 6 weeks after creation. Radiology 279(2):620–629

Salgado O, Chacón R, Henríquez C (2004) Ulnar-basilic fistula: indications, surgical aspects, puncture technique, and results. Artif Organs 28(7):634–638

Schmidli J, Widmer M, Basile C, de Donato G, Gallieni M, Gibbons C et al (2018) Editor's Choice – Vascular Access: 2018 Clinical Practice Guidelines of the European Society for Vascular Surgery (ESVS). Eur J Vasc Endovasc Surg 55(6):757–818

Sha H, Luk T, Tee S, Hardin R, Seak C (2016) Our experience in using the brachial venae comitantes as a native vascular access for hemodialysis. Hemodial Int 20(2):293–297

Sharma S, Bera S, Goyal V, Gupta V, Bisht N (2021) Ulnar-basilic arteriovenous fistula for hemodialysis access: utility as the "second procedure" after radio cephalic fistula. Ann Vasc Dis 14(2):132–138

Siracuse J, Cheng T, Arinze N, Levin S, Jones D, Malas M et al (2019) Snuffbox arteriovenous fistulas have similar outcomes and patency as wrist arteriovenous fistulas. J Vasc Surg 70(2):554–561

Teixeira G, Almeida P, Sousa C, Teles P, Sousa P, Loureiro L et al (2017) Arteriovenous access banding revisited. J Vasc Access 18(3):225–231

Uzun H, Çiçek O, Seren M (2019) Transposition of basilic vein in forearm for arteriovenous fistula creation: our mid-term results. Turk Gogus Kalp Damar Cerrahisi Derg 27(4):508–511

Vascular Access 2006 Work Croup (2006) Clinical practice guidelines for vascular access. Am J Kidney Dis 48(Suppl 1):S176–S247

Voorzaat B, van der Bogt K, Janmaat C, van Schaik J, Dekker F, Rotmans J (2018) Arteriovenous fistula maturation failure in a large cohort of hemodialysis patients in the Netherlands. World J Surg 42(6):1895–1903

Wong V, Ward R, Taylor J, Selvakumar S, How T, Bakran A (1996) Factors associated with early failure of arteriovenous fistulae for haemodialysis access. Eur J Vasc Endovasc Surg 12(2):207–213

Physical Examination of the Arteriovenous Fistula

Nurten Ozen and Clemente Neves Sousa

Physical examination of an arteriovenous fistula (AVF) can be easily carried out and is a cost-effective method that can be performed with little equipment in a short period of time. The examination purpose is to extend the duration of the vascular access by detecting in advance any dysfunction or complications related to the AVF (Salman and Beathard 2013; Sousa et al. 2013; Lok et al. 2020). Failure to detect dysfunction in a timely manner leads to an increase in morbidity and mortality due to the development of aneurysms, hematomas, thrombosis, and inappropriate dialysis in AVF (Lok et al. 2020; Sidawy et al. 2008).

Physical examination of the AVF should be conducted systematically (Fig. 1) and it is carried out by using three methods: inspection, palpation, and auscultation. Guidelines recommend the examination to be regularly performed by the patient, nurse, and nephrologist (Ibeas et al. 2017; Lok et al. 2020; Sidawy et al. 2008; Schmidli et al. 2018; Harduin et al. 2023). The patient should daily perform inspection, palpation, and the arm elevation test; the nurse should perform inspection, palpation, auscultation, and the arm elevation test during each dialysis session; the nephrologist should perform inspection, palpation, auscultation, arm elevation, and pulse augmentation tests once a month and when an issue is identified (Ibeas et al. 2017; Schmidli et al. 2018; Abreo et al. 2019; Norton de Matos et al. 2023). The physical examination is divided into a summary assessment and a systematic assessment. The purpose of the

---

N. Ozen (✉)
Faculty of Nursing, Department of Internal Medicine Nursing, Istanbul University, Istanbul, Turkey
e-mail: nurten.ozen@istanbul.edu.tr

C. N. Sousa
Nursing School of University of Porto, Porto, Portugal
e-mail: clementesousa@esenf.pt

RISE – Health, University of Porto, Porto, Portugal

© The Author(s), under exclusive license to Springer Nature Switzerland AG 2025
N. Ozen et al. (eds.), *Arteriovenous Fistula Management*,
https://doi.org/10.1007/978-3-032-04771-7_3

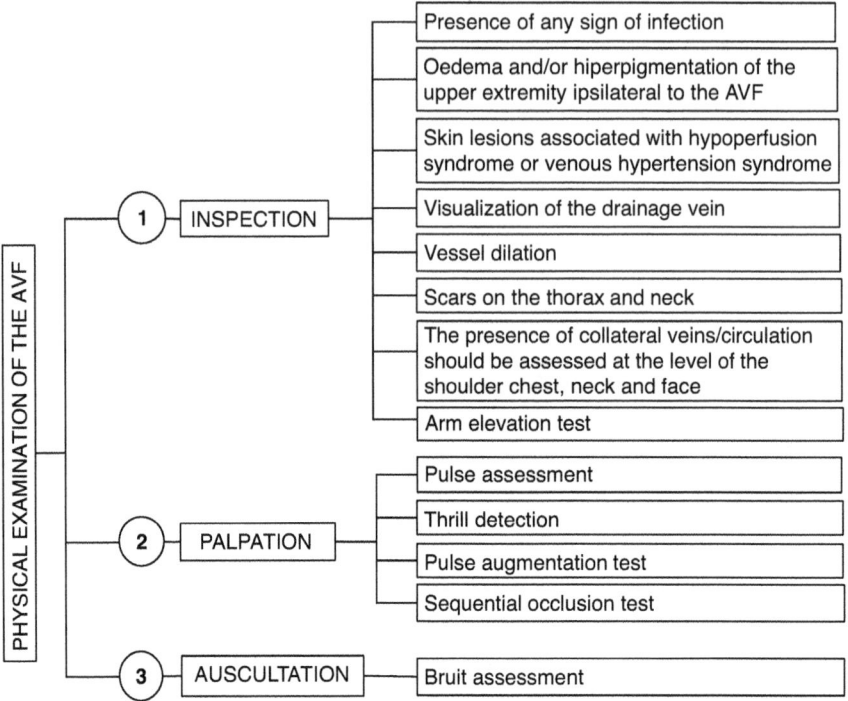

Fig. 1 Physical examination of the AVF

summary assessment is to determine whether the AVF is appropriate for cannulation and the initiation of hemodialysis treatment. The systematic assessment focuses on identifying any issues or complications associated with the AVF.

1 Inspection

The inspection corresponds to observing the arm of the AVF, including the thorax, and should compare the arm with the contra-lateral arm. Observing the region where the AVF is located is of utmost importance. Additionally, the diameter of the vein, the presence of collaterals, and the shoulder, chest, breast, and neck area of the other extremity should also be examined. Attention should be paid to any signs of infection, as the infection can be either superficial or deep (Abreo et al. 2019). Cannulation-related superficial infections can develop, while deep infections exhibit classic signs and symptoms of infection such as redness, tenderness, swelling, and purulent discharge (Abreo et al. 2019; Lok et al. 2020; Salman and Beathard 2013; Ibeas et al. 2017; Schmidli et al. 2018; Pinto et al. 2022).

The presence of collateral veins in the arm or chest should be carefully checked, as it indicates downstream stenosis. Patients should be monitored for the presence of aneurysms and pseudoaneurysms (Norton de Matos et al. 2023). Skin thinning, decreased pigmentation, ulceration, or spontaneous bleeding should be checked in patients and recorded in their file. When the overlying skin becomes as thin as tissue paper and cannot be grasped between the index finger and thumb, it is a likely sign of an aneurysm and may require prompt intervention (Abreo et al. 2019; Lok et al. 2020; Salman and Beathard 2013). Through inspection, symptoms related to distal hyperfusion, which causes ischemia in the hand, can also be observed in patients. The affected hand may appear pale and cyanotic compared to the opposite side, and in severe cases, color changes and ulcers can be seen at the fingertips (Abreo et al. 2019; Lok et al. 2020; Salman and Beathard 2013).

Arm Elevation Test or Fistula Collapse Test

The arm elevation or fistula collapse test allows the assessment of the existence of outflow problems, mainly stenosis in the vein draining the fistula. It should be routinely carried out during AVF inspection and should be considered part of the physical examination (Salman and Beathard 2013; Sousa et al. 2013; Ibeas et al. 2017).

This test consists of raising the patient's access arm above the level of the heart, with expected fistula collapse (Sharma and Niyyar 2021). Even if the patient has a large, dilated AVF, it should remain flaccid when the arm containing the fistula is raised. In the presence of stenosis, blood drainage is impaired and the AVF does not collapse. The vein remains full, firm to the touch, and there is no collapse of the anastomosis with the stenosis after the vein collapses (Salman and Beathard 2013; Norton de Matos et al. 2023).

It is a simple, noninvasive, quick, and low-cost test that can be easily taught and used by nephrologists, nephrology nurses, dialysis professionals, and even patients themselves in order to rule out stenosis (Sousa et al. 2014; Vachharajani et al. 2015; Ibeas et al. 2017).

2 Palpation

Following inspection, physical examination should continue with palpation. Palpation involves the assessment of two important indicators: pulse and thrill. This helps in detecting any fistula dysfunction. During palpation, additional maneuvers like pulse augmentation and sequential occlusion should also be carried out (Sousa et al. 2013; Ibeas et al. 2017).

The pulse in the fistula is assessed with two fingers. There is one normal pulse and two pathological pulses associated with the AVF (Salman and Beathard 2013; Abreo et al. 2019):

- Normal pulse: it is soft and can be easily felt with slight pressure. It represents appropriate drainage through the vein without problems.

- Hypopulsatile pulse: it is characterized by being weak and easy to compress. It is an anomaly that usually indicates the presence of a stenotic lesion in the inflow. The problems can be in the feeding artery, the anastomosis, or the juxta-anastomosis.
- Hyperpulsatile pulse: it is characterized by a strong pulse that is difficult to compress. It is a disfunction that generally indicates problems with the outflow, usually stenosis.

The degree of pulsation provides a clue as to the severity and location of the stenosis (Sousa et al. 2013). In the case of inflow stenosis, the pulse is hypopulsatile and the result of the pulse-increase test is hypopulsatile. In the case of outflow stenosis, the pulse is hyperpulsatile up to the site of the stenosis, after which there is a weak or absent pulse (Salman and Beathard 2013; Sharma and Niyyar 2021).

The thrill is a vibration felt with the palm of the hand and provides information about the blood flow circulating along the artery. In the case of a fistula, the thrill should be continuous (both during systole and diastole) (Sousa et al. 2013; Abreo et al. 2019). There are two types of thrill that can be observed in a fistula:

- Normal thrill: a soft, continuous and diffuse baseline vibration characteristic of a well-functioning. This finding is typically appreaciable along the entire course of the AVF, with maximal intensity at the anastomotic site and progressive attenuation along the venous segment.
- Abnormal thrill: the vibration may be confined to the anastomotic region, may exhibit discontinuity (with intervening segments devoid of thrill), or may be detectable in the shoulder and/or axillary regions. In some cases, the thrill may be entirely absent.

The absence of a thrill indicates that there is no blood flow in the fistula. If the thrill is diminished, it suggests the presence of inflow stenosis, while an increased thrill points to outflow stenosis (Salman and Beathard 2013; Norton de Matos et al. 2023). If both thrill and pulse are absent at the same time, it indicates thrombosis in the AVF.

Pulse Augmentation Test

The pulse augmentation test is used to analyze the inflow, typically detecting stenosis (Sousa et al. 2013). This test is carried out by occluding the access several centimeters above the arterial anastomosis with one finger while assessing the intensity of the pulse with the other finger. An increase in pressure occurs before the point at which pressure is applied and the pulse becomes hyperpulsatile. In such a situation, the pulse is normal.

If problems occur anywhere in the arterial system, from the anastomosis upwards, they will affect the passage of blood into the venous system, with implications for the pulse (Sharma and Niyyar 2021; Ibeas et al. 2017; Abreo et al. 2019). When performing the pulse augmentation test, the pulse is hypopulsatile and therefore abnormal, indicating an inflow problem. The degree of this increase in pulse intensity is directly proportional to the quality of the access stream (Salman and Beathard 2013; Sousa et al. 2014).

Sequential Occlusion Test

This test is similar to the pulse augmentation test but is focused on the disappearance of the pulsation sensation when the vein connected to the artery in the AVF is temporarily blocked. The aim of the test is to identify the side branches that extend from the fistula.

It is a test that involves blocking the draining vein closest to the connection point with one finger while simultaneously feeling the usual pulsation sensation over the connection point with the other hand, based on the relationship between vein vibration and blood flow (Salman and Beathard 2013; Sharma and Niyyar 2021; Ibeas et al. 2017). The pulsing sensation, usually detectable at the arterial connection point which indicates blood flow, disappears when the vein is manually occluded upstream, causing a temporary interruption in blood flow. The entire length of the vein should then be examined, gradually moving the point of obstruction upwards. If the sensation of pulsation is still present at any point along the vein, it suggests the presence of collateral flow distal to the occlusion point (Salman and Beathard 2013; Norton de Matos et al. 2023).

3 Auscultation

A continuous bruit can be heard during systole and diastole in a normal fistula. The auscultation phase involves listening to the normal bruit and recognizing any changes that may occur. When there is a narrowing (stenosis) in the blood vessel, it leads to a distinct sound known as bruit (Sousa et al. 2013; Ibeas et al. 2017; Abreo et al. 2019). This sound is characterized by a high-pitched noise mainly during the systolic phase of the heartbeat. The bruit is more pronounced downstream of the stenosis, indicating turbulent blood flow caused by narrowing (Salman and Beathard 2013). There are two distinct types of bruit that can be heard:

- Normal bruit: the normal auscultatory finding of an AVF consists of a continuous. low-frequency systolic-diastolic bruit, indicative of laminar and stable blood flow throughout the entire draining vein. This uninterrupted acoustic pattern is typically audible throughout the vein's course, in segments wherw haemodynamic conditions remain unchanged and free of stenosis obstructions (Sousa et al. 2014; Ibeas et al. 2017).
- Abnormal bruit: an abnormal bruit is generally predominantly systolic and arises from haemodynamically significant turbulent flow as blood traverses a stenosis segment of the draining vein. Clinically, it is characterized by a higher-pitched

anf more wheezing or whistling sound, which becomes more pronounced during systole, coinciding with the increase in velocities at the site of narrowing (Salman and Beathard 2013; Sharma and Niyyar 2022).

4 Practical Implications

Physical examination is a noninvasive method that can be quickly conducted, is cost-effective, is practical, and provides valuable assistance in the diagnosis. Proper management of the vascular access route in patients undergoing hemodialysis treatment ensures that the patient derives maximum benefit from treatment. It also reduces morbidity and mortality rates. Accurate physical examination enables the detection of fistula dysfunction, allowing timely intervention to extend the lifespan of both the fistula and the patient. Therefore, it is of utmost importance for experienced healthcare professionals to perform physical examinations during every dialysis session of patients undergoing hemodialysis treatment in order to identify stenosis and fistula dysfunction.

References

Abreo K, Amin B, Abreo A (2019) Physical examination of the hemodialysis arteriovenous fistula to detect early dysfunction. J Vasc Access 20(1):7–11

Harduin L, Barroso TGJ, Filippo M, Almeida L, Castro-Santos G, Oliveira J (2023) Guidelines on vascular access for hemodialysis from the Brazilian Society of Angiology and Vascular Surgery. J Vasc Bras 30(22):e20230052. https://doi.org/10.1590/1677-5449.202300522

Ibeas J, Roca-Tey R, Vallespín J, Moreno T, Moñux G, Martí-Monrós A et al (2017) Spanish clinical guidelines on vascular access for haemodialysis. Nefrologia 37(Suppl 1):1–191

Lok CE, Huber TS, Lee T, Shenoy S, Yevzlin AS, Abreo K et al (2020) National Kidney Foundation. KDOQI Clinical Practice Guideline for Vascular Access: 2019 Update. Am J Kidney Dis 75(4 Suppl 2):S1–S164. https://doi.org/10.1053/j.ajkd.2019.12.001. Epub 2020 Mar 12. Erratum in: Am J Kidney Dis (2021) 77(4):551

Norton de Matos A, Sousa C, Teixiera G (2023) Doppler Ultrasound in vascular access for haemodialysis. Gráfica de Paredes, Lda, Porto

Pinto R, Sousa C, Salgueiro A, Fernandes I (2022) Arteriovenous fistula cannulation in hemodialysis: a vascular access clinical practice guidelines narrative review. J Vasc Access 23(5):825–831

Salman L, Beathard G (2013) Interventional nephrology: physical examination as a tool for surveillance for the hemodialysis arteriovenous access. Clin J Am Soc Nephrol 8(7):1220–1227

Schmidli J, Widmer M, Basile C, de Donato G, Gallieni M, Gibbons C et al (2018) Editor's choice - vascular access: 2018 clinical practice guidelines of the European Society for Vascular Surgery (ESVS). Eur J Vasc Endovasc Surg 55(6):757–818

Sharma M, Niyyar V (2021) Evaluation of suspected outflow stenosis in an aneurysmal AVF. Kidney 360 2(6):1072–1073

Sharma MK, Niyyar VD (2022) Preoperative evaluation: physical examination. In: Yevzlin AS, Asif A, Salman L, Ramani K, Qaqish SS, Vachharajani TJ (eds.) Interventional nephrology: principles and practice. 2nd edn. Springer, Switzerland, pp 7–17

Sidawy AN, Spergel LM, Besarab A, Allon M, Jennings WC, Padberg FT Jr et al (2008) The Society for Vascular Surgery: clinical practice guidelines for the surgical placement and maintenance of arteriovenous hemodialysis access. J Vasc Surg 48(5 Suppl):2S–25S. https://doi.org/10.1016/j.jvs.2008.08.042

Sousa C, Apóstolo J, Figueiredo M, Martins M, Dias V (2013) Physical examination: how to examine the arm with arteriovenous fistula. Hemodial Int 17(2):300–306

Sousa C, Teles P, Dias V, Apóstolo J, Figueiredo M, Martins M (2014) Physical examination of arteriovenous fistula: the influence of professional experience in the detection of complications. Hemodial Int 18(3):695–699

Vachharajani TJ, Wu S, Brouwer-Maier D, Asif A (2015) Arteriovenous fistulas and grafts: the basics. In: Daugirdas JT, Blake PG, Ing TS (eds) Handbook of dialysis, 5th edn. Wolters Kluwer Health, United States, pp 99–120

Arteriovenous Fistula Complications

Nurten Ozen, Clemente Neves Sousa, and Tayfun Eyileten

The arteriovenous fistula (AVF) is considered by the scientific community as the best vascular access when compared to a graft or a central venous catheter. The risk of infectious complications at the initiation of haemodialysis (HD) is four times higher when a central venous catheter is used compared to an AVF (Lok and Foley 2013). The morbidity and mortality of patients undergoing HD are directly correlated with the type of vascular access chosen (Ibeas et al. 2017). Furthermore, multiple complications that can compromise patency and affect the effectiveness of treatment may occur with an AVF.

Thus, detection and treatment of complications at an early stage is key in order to prevent escalation to more serious illnesses. Their identification followed by an appropriate intervention lead to cost reduction and shorter hospital stays.

N. Ozen (✉)
Faculty of Nursing, Department of Internal Medicine Nursing, Istanbul University, Istanbul, Turkey
e-mail: nurten.ozen@istanbul.edu.tr

C. N. Sousa
Nursing School of University of Porto, Porto, Portugal
e-mail: clementesousa@esenf.pt

RISE – Health, University of Porto, Porto, Portugal

T. Eyileten
Guven Hospital, Department of Nephrology, Ankara, Turkey
e-mail: teyileten@gmail.com

© The Author(s), under exclusive license to Springer Nature Switzerland AG 2025
N. Ozen et al. (eds.), *Arteriovenous Fistula Management*,
https://doi.org/10.1007/978-3-032-04771-7_4

1 Stenosis

Stenosis is the AVF main complication and can compromise its functionality and HD effectiveness. A number of vascular access guidelines define the required criteria to rate a stenosis as significant (Kukita et al. 2015; Schmidli et al. 2018; Lok et al. 2020). Stenosis is typically defined as a reduction of more than 50% in the lumen. However, the Spanish vascular access guidelines have defined primary criteria (>50% reduction in diameter and two to three times increase in maximum systolic velocity) and additional criteria (residual diameter <1.9 to 2.0 mm; >25% reduction in flow; and flow <500 ml/min) (Ibeas et al. 2017; Norton de Matos et al. 2023). These guidelines introduce the concept of borderline stenosis and significant stenosis. Borderline stenosis is when only the primary criteria are present and requires surveillance. Significant stenosis occurs when the primary criteria are present and one of the additional criteria is also present. In such a situation, stenosis must be intervened upon (Ibeas et al. 2017). Hence, only stenoses that cause a hemodynamic effect (leading to a decrease in the lumen area by $\geq 70\%$) and are associated with reduced flow, elevated venous pressures, prolonged time to haemostasis, or abnormal physical examination findings (such as diminished thrill or pulsatile flow) should be considered for treatment (Schmidli et al. 2018).

Clinical suspicion of stenosis is confirmed by the presence of a number of factors, including reduced dialysis quality and issues with needling, such as prolonged bleeding after AVF puncture, localized pain around the fistula, or elevated venous pressure (Sousa et al. 2013; Pinto et al. 2022, 2024). Recirculation stands as a crucial concern due to its substantial role in causing inadequate HD. The primary culprit often lies in the presence of high-grade venous stenosis, which obstructs the venous outflow, consequently causing a backflow into the arterial needle. Diagnosis of recirculation occurs when dialyzed blood returning through the venous side reenters the dialyzer via the arterial needle, rather than returning to the systemic circulation. Ultrasound plays a key role in detecting AVF stenosis, being a noninvasive, safe, and accessible tool. It enables directly assessing blood flow in real time and identifying changes in the vessels' structure (Norton de Matos et al. 2023). Moreover, ultrasound enables measuring flow velocity and detecting abnormal patterns that indicate the presence of stenosis. This helps identifying the correct time for intervention (Norton de Matos et al. 2023).

Based on its location, an AVF can be ranked into the following three categories, enabling a more accurate assessment of the AVF and better understanding of stenosis and its clinical behavior (Norton de Matos et al. 2023):

- Inflow: it is considered from the aortic valve to the pre-cannulation vein, including the artery, anastomosis, and the juxta-anastomotic segment. These vascular lesions are located in the feeder artery that supplies blood to the vascular access. The resulting haemodynamic disruption manifests primarily as a reduction in AVF flow. This reduction is primarily attributed to the development of stenotic or occlusive lesions that result from the advancement of preexisting underlying atherosclerosis. Meanwhile, anastomosis and juxta-anastomotic segment problems arise from technical complications during the creation of the anastomosis. This

Table 1 Characteristic sites of stenosis and corresponding advantages and disadvantages

Access type	Common site of stenosis	Advantages	Disadvantages
Distal access (snuffbox; radiocephalic; ulnarbasilic fistula)	Inflow (anastomosis or juxta-anastomosis)	Ease of creation, preservation of the upstream vein for future access creation	Longer maturation time and a lower flow rate
Proximal access (brachiocephalic fistula)	Outflow (cephalic arch or swing segment)	Ease of creation, high flow rates, high rate of maturation	Increased incidence of steal syndrome, increased risk of ischemic monomelic neuropathy, and higher rates of symptomatic central venous stenosis
Transposition (brachiobasilic or brachiobrachial fistula)	Outflow (transition to depth, in the swing segment)	High flow rates, high rate of maturation	Two surgeries are required and are associated with an increased risk of steal syndrome, increased occurrence of ischemic monomelic neuropathy, and elevated rates of symptomatic central venous stenosis

stenosis causes a weakened thrill, cannulation challenges, reduced flows, and elevated negative arterial pressures.

- Midflow: It corresponds to the venous segment between the arterial cannulation and the venous cannulation used in the AVF. Clinically, it is characterized by an increased pulse and signs such as a prolonged haemostasis time after needle removal, difficulty in needling, and increased venous pressure during the dialysis session.
- Outflow: it is considered from the vein after the site of venous cannulation until the right atrium. It prompts the fistula to exhibit tension, pulsation, and aneurysmal growth. Higher venous pressures become apparent during dialysis. Both inflow and outflow stenosis result in compromised access flows, potentially leading to access thrombosis.

Characteristic sites of stenosis and corresponding advantages and disadvantages are provided in Table 1 (Quencer and Arici 2015; Quencer et al. 2017).

2 Hemodialysis access-induced distal ischemia

Hemodialysis access–induced distal ischemia (HAIDI) is connected to both AVFs and dialysis access grafts, causing reduced arterial pressure and compromised perfusion in the hand. The extent of ischemic complications varies widely (Kmentova et al. 2018). The incidence of occurrence in patients varies between 1% and 8% (Beathard and Spergel 2013) according to the literature. However, approximately 5% experience this condition once in their lifetime (Padberg et al. 2008). The incidence of HAIDI will rise due to the frequent use of autogenous elbow fistulas, a type of access that is associated with chronic ischemia (Kmentova et al. 2018).

Certain clinical conditions such as peripheral vascular disease, diabetes mellitus, advanced age, the use of the brachial artery for anastomosis, multiple previous vascular access procedures, female gender, high access blood flow, and a history of amputation are identified as factors that can increase the risk of developing HAIDI (Beathard et al. 2020).

Symptoms are often of moderate severity, but can occasionally be severe and deteriorate rapidly (Table 2). HAIDI may occur as a result of previous arterial disease or by a phenomenon of steal hemodynamics associated with a high blood-flow access (Teixeira et al. 2021; Norton de Matos et al. 2023). In the former situation, the AVF has a normal flow or a low output but the existence of an arterial stenosis can compromise distal circulation. Such a kind of HAIDI is usually found in elderly people and those with diabetes or other arteriosclerotic diseases. When the problem can no longer be solved by endovascular treatment, access ligation can be considered. The latter situation arises when the AVF has high blood flow and such an excess flow will cause signs and symptoms associated with distal ischemia. This mechanism may be aggravated by insufficient vascular adaptive changes, vasospasm, or failure in compensatory vasodilation of the arterial network, culminating in tissue hypoperfusion and ischemic symptoms, especially in high-flow brachial accesses (Teixeira et al. 2021).

Table 2 Clinical classification of HAIDI

Stage	Signs and symptoms
I	• No clear symptoms, only signs • Nail beds slightly cyanotic and/or pale, mild coldness of skin of hand, decreased pulse at wrist
IIa	• Nail beds cyanotic or pale, coldness of skin of hand, decreased pulse at wrist • Tolerable pain, cramps, paresthesia, numbness during dialysis or with exercise of hand
IIb	• Nail beds cyanotic or pale, coldness of skin of hand, decreased pulse at wrist • Intolerable pain, cramps, paresthesia, numbness during dialysis or with exercise of hand
III	• Nail beds cyanotic or pale, coldness of skin of hand, decreased pulse at wrist • Rest pain or motor dysfunction of fingers or hand
IVa	• Tissue loss such as ulceration, necrosis • Motor and/or sensory loss
IVb	• Extensive tissue loss

In these cases, the techniques used associated with flow reduction allow ischemia to be corrected (Teixeira et al. 2017; Norton de Matos et al. 2023).

A patient with symptoms compatible with HAIDI should undergo a comprehensive clinical examination. First, the patient's comorbidity status should be addressed, and their frailty assessed. HAIDI diagnosis shortens the expected lifespan of the patient, thus making it important for clinical assessment to be carried out by the nurse before each dialysis session (Tonelli et al. 2015). Clinical classification plays a significant role in determining the management of HAIDI. For a patient in Stage I and IIa, warm application can be done using a glove or a water bag filled with warm water, and hand exercises can be recommended. For patients in other stages, surgical interventions may be required (Scheltinga et al. 2009).

Diagnosis is usually made based on symptoms and angiography and/or ultrasound. Clinical signs such as skin coldness, pallor, cyanosis, decreased sensation, and ultimately, ulceration and even gangrene can be observed. Therefore, conducting a physical examination of the hand is important. Radial and ulnar pulses are usually diminished or absent, but rarely, despite clinical signs and symptoms, pulses can be normal. A decrease in capillary refill time, an indicator of decreased peripheral perfusion, also aids in diagnosing the condition. A capillary refill time of less than 3 seconds indicates good peripheral perfusion, while a time exceeding 5 seconds signifies an abnormality (Inston et al. 2017a; Beathard et al. 2020). With regard to ultrasound diagnosis, the identification of high-access blood flow or arterial pathology (in many cases with the aid of angiography) enables the best therapeutic strategy to be adapted (Teixeira et al. 2021).

3 Steal Syndrome

Syndrome is a relatively common side effect of having an AVF, with a reported prevalence of up to 8% in the population undergoing hemodialysis, and increasing to between 75% and 90% in groups at risk (elderly patients, patients with diabetes, and peripheral vascular disease) (Stolic 2013).

HAIDI symptomatology is similar to that observed in other ischemic conditions, including pain at rest, paresthesias, weakness or paralysis, absence of distal pulses, skin pallor, and sensation of cold, resulting from arterial hypoperfusion of the distal tissues. In more severe instances, it can progress to tissue necrosis and irreversible loss. Patients may exhibit pale/bluish and/or cold hands, painless/with pain during exercise and/or HD, ischemic pain at rest, ulceration, necrosis and gangrene (Stolic 2013), diminished or absent radial and ulnar pulses, relieve of symptoms when compressing the arteriovenous access, ischemic changes, brachial artery digital index of 0.6 or less, digital pressures below 50 mmHg or non-recordable, and abnormal waveform suggestive of steal (Malik et al. 2008).

Presence of diabetes mellitus, use of the brachial artery, peripheral arteriopathy, advanced age, smoking, female sex, and history of vascular access failures in the same limb are considered as risk factors for the development of ischemia (Scali and Huber 2011; Lok et al. 2020).

A well-developed AVF, especially when it exhibits a high flow, can divert a significant portion of blood flow to the vein, compromising distal perfusion. This relative hypoperfusion can manifest clinically as severe pain, hand coldness, and changes in skin color such as pallor or cyanosis. The pulse is often weak or absent and neuropathic features may manifest with time, culminating in a typical "claw hand" contracture (Lok et al. 2020).

Patients with highly abnormal baseline distal circulation should be considered at high risk for steal syndrome. They can have conventional access constructions performed but their hand perfusion should be monitored closely thereafter in order to prevent irreversible ischemic changes in the digits. Although the most serious sign of steal is gangrene, patients may develop small nonhealing ulcers at the sites of fingersticks for glucose testing, digital stiffness, paronychias, or severe pain (Teixeira et al. 2021). If these changes occur, the patient should have urgent conversion of the access site to a different configuration or access ligation (Kaufman 2017; Lok et al. 2020).

Although insufficient flow is problematic because it leads to thrombosis of the access construction, a more dangerous and increasingly common problem is steal, which can lead to significant dysfunction or damage in the affected extremity. In order for steal to occur, three factors must be present: disease in the inflow arteries, such that they cannot dilate to meet access flow demands; disease in the distal vessels, such that they have higher than normal resistance to flow; and a low-resistance access construction conduit (Teixeira et al. 2017). Symptoms can range from a hand that is cold or numb only during treatments, to mononeuropathy with intrinsic muscle weakness in the hand, to rest pain in the extremity with gangrene. The diagnosis of the steal phenomenon is only possible at the bedside with a Doppler. If occlusion causes flow to increase, especially if it goes from none to vigorous with visible hyperemia of digits, the diagnosis is certain. For minor steal, the access site can be followed, reserving repair or revision for the patient who does not demonstrate adaptation to the symptoms. For major steal that threatens the limb, an urgent procedure is appropriate (Kaufman 2017; Lok et al. 2020).

The diagnosis of steal syndrome is associated with changes in the nails, occasional tingling, coldness in the extremities, tingling and numbness in the hands and fingers, muscle weakness, pale to whitish or cyanotic nail beds, pain at rest, deficits in sensory and motor function, ulcerations, and necrosis of the fingertips. The most common symptoms associated with theft occur in the mild and severe stages of the disease (Malik et al. 2008; Norton de Matos et al. 2023). The accurate way to diagnose the presence of steal syndrome is through ultrasound, because when inversion of the distal flow occurs, there is anastomosis (Norton de Matos et al. 2023).

4 Infection

The incidence of arteriovenous-access infections is relatively low, particularly for AVFs. Infection may be identified as an area with pain, heat, and redness or as a small abscess or scar in the needling area (Ibeas et al. 2017) and accounts for about 20% of all complications associated with AVFs (Stolic 2013). In the Al-Jaishi's systematic review, the median infection rates per 1000 patient days was 0.11 (16 cohorts; $n = 6439$ fistulas) (Al-Jaishi 2017). This kind of complication can vary in terms of severity, ranging from localized cellulitis (redness) to the formation of abscesses (swelling and tenderness), and even bacteremia (fever and weakness). Many cases arise from needle punctures and the incidence of perioperative infection after the creation of a fistula is approximately 5%.

When complications with an AVF arise, infection is a major clinical problem, often leading to hospitalization and increased mortality (Collins et al. 2013). The incidence of AVF infection is usually low, but may be influenced by the type of cannulation technique used. For instance, buttonhole cannulation may increase the risk of infection (Muir et al. 2014; Christensen et al. 2018). The underlying mechanisms responsible for the development of arteriovenous access infections are likely to be multifactorial and include both patient- and system-related issues. Skin organisms *Staphylococcus aureus* and *Staphylococcus epidermidis* account for 70%–90% of arteriovenous access infections (Lafrance et al. 2008) in the upper extremity, with a higher incidence of Gram-negative organisms in lower-extremity AV accesses (Schneider et al. 2012).

Patients with arteriovenous access infections require timely detection, diagnosis, and treatment to prevent poor outcomes. Visible signs and symptoms range from mild cellulitis around the cannulation site to bacteremia and overwhelming sepsis. Physical examination and routine laboratory studies are usually sufficient to establish the diagnosis. However, additional imaging can help corroborate the diagnosis and define the extent of arteriovenous access involvement. In particular, duplex ultrasound can be used to confirm patency, examine the integrity of the arteriovenous access wall, confirm the presence of any aneurysms/pseudoaneurysms, document the presence of fluid around the vein/nonautogenous access, and help determine the extent of the infection (Legout et al. 2012; Sousa et al. 2013). Other imaging studies can be used, including CT, PET, indium scans, and technetium scans, although they are rarely necessary and not as universally available (Legout et al. 2012). Oral or intravenous antibiotic treatment is generally successful in such cases (Siddiky et al. 2014).

5 Aneurysms

The systematic review by Al-Jaishi reports median aneurysm rates of 0.04 per 1000 patient days (14 unique cohorts; $n = 1827$ fistulas) (Al-Jaishi 2017). The incidence of aneurysm varies between 5% and 60% (Stolic 2013) and its prevalence in the HD population is over 40%. It is characterized by the widening of all three layers of the vessel wall, with a diameter greater than 18 mm. The natural progression of aneurysms in the vascular access is not well defined. Even though classifications for these aneurysms exist, they are not consistently used in research or clinical settings.

The precise mechanism behind the development of aneurysmal dilation remains unknown but it seems to result from a combination of excessive external remodeling, changes in the vessel wall due to injury, and outflow problems. The diagnosis of arteriovenous access aneurysms relies on physical examination and ultrasound. Venography and cross-sectional imaging might also be necessary, particularly in the investigation of outflow obstructions.

In patients with outflow stenosis, the AVF wall may weaken over time due to increased intra-access pressure, leading to expansion and to the development of an aneurysm (Norton de Matos et al. 2023). Aneurysms are more likely to develop in areas where the vessel wall is weakened, especially due to repeated cannulations in the same location. Generalized and progressive degeneration of all AVFs or at some sites makes the skin more fragile, increasing the time of hemostasis or bleeding, infection and ulceration (Stolic 2013). Occurrence of spots or ulcerations is a vascular emergency and the patient should be quickly referred to a vascular surgeon. The dialysis team should implement a vascular access monitoring and surveillance program, including the assessment for aneurysms (Sousa et al. 2024).

Aneurysm repair is recommended when symptomatic complications arise or when aneurysms grow to a size that affects the patient's quality of life or the use of the AVF (such as skin changes like thinning, pain, thrombosis, venous hypertension, or shortened area for cannulation) (Pasklinsky et al. 2011). Surgical intervention is recommended when there is a risk of rupture and ulceration of the aneurysm, presence of bleeding elements, or when there is limited space for puncture due to the size of the aneurysm (Wiese and Nonnast-Daniel 2004).

Pseudoaneurysm, on the other hand, is a rupture of the layers of the vein and usually results from a leak originating from an orifice, often due to iatrogenic trauma, especially from repeated needle punctures (Saeed et al. 2011). Treatment of pseudoaneurysms in fistulas with smaller diameter ruptures can be done by resealing this site. When the size of the vein rupture is very large, placement of a polytetrafluoroethylene (PTFE) segment may be necessary. These situations lack an evidence-based approach and depend on clinical experience and available medical resources (Inston et al. 2017b).

6 Practical Implications

All patients with an AVF need to be monitored for the emergence of signs and symptoms of complications. Once a diagnosis of complication has been established, the patient should undergo a comprehensive clinical assessment to determine the suitable management approach.

References

Al-Jaishi AL (2017) Complications of the arteriovenous fistula: a systematic review. J Am Soc Nephrol 28 (6):1839–1850

Beathard G, Spergel L (2013) Hand ischemia associated with dialysis vascular access: an individualized access flow-based approach to therapy. Semin Dial 26 (3):287–314

Beathard G, Jennings W, Wasse H, Shenoy S, Hentschel DM, Abreo K et al (2020) ASDIN white paper: Assessment and management of hemodialysis access-induced distal ischemia by interventional nephrologists. J Vasc Access 21 (5):543–553

Christensen L, Skadborg M, Mortensen A, Mortensen C, Møller J, Lemming L et al (2018) Bacteriology of the buttonhole cannulation tract in hemodialysis patients: a prospective cohort study. Am J Kidney Dis 72 (2):234–242

Collins A, Foley R, Herzog C, Chavers B, Gilbertson D, Herzog C et al (2013) US Renal Data System 2012 Annual Data Report. Am J Kidney Dis 61 (1 Suppl 1):A7, e1–476

Ibeas J, Roca-Tey R, Vallespín J, Moreno T, Moñux G, Martí-Monrós A et al (2017) Spanish Clinical Guidelines on vascular access for haemodialysis. Nefrologia 37 (Suppl 1):1–191

Inston N, Mistry H, Gilbert J, Kingsmore D, Raza Z, Tozzi M et al (2017) Aneurysms in vascular access: state of the art and future developments. J Vasc Access 18 (6):464–472

Inston N, Schanzer H, Widmer M, Deane C, Wilkins J, Davidson I et al (2017) Arteriovenous access ischemic steal (AVAIS) in haemodialysis: a consensus from the Charing Cross Vascular Access Masterclass 2016. J Vasc Access 18 (1):3–12

Kaufman J (2017) Noninfectious complications from vascular access. In: Nisseson EA, Fine R, Mehrotra R, Zaritsky J (eds.). Handbook of dialysis therapy. Elsevier, Philadelphia, pp 50–63

Kmentova T, Valerianova A, Kovarova L, Lachmanova J, Hladinova Z, Malik J (2018) Decrease of muscle strength in vascular access hand due to silent ischaemia. J Vasc Access 19 (6):573–577

Kukita K, Ohira S, Amano I, Naito H, Azuma N, Ikeda K et al (2015) 2011 update Japanese Society for Dialysis Therapy Guidelines of Vascular Access Construction and Repair for Chronic Hemodialysis. Ther Apher Dial 19 (Suppl 1):1–39

Lafrance J, Rahme E, Lelorier J, Iqbal S (2008) Vascular access-related infections: definitions, incidence rates, and risk factors. Am J Kidney Dis 52 (5):982–993

Legout L, D'Elia P, Sarraz-Bournet B, Haulon S, Meybeck A, Senneville E et al (2012) Diagnosis and management of prosthetic vascular graft infections. Med Mal Infect 42 (3):102–109

Lok C, Foley R (2013) Vascular access morbidity and mortality: trends of the last decade. Clin J Am Soc Nephrol 8 (7):1213–1219

Lok C, Huber T, Lee T, Shenoy S, Yevzlin A, Abreo K et al (2020) KDOQI Vascular Access Guideline Work Group. KDOQI clinical practice guideline for vascular access: 2019 update. Am J Kidney Dis 75 (4 Suppl 2):S1–S164

Malik J, Tuka V, Kasalova Z, Chytilova E, Slavikova M, Clagett P et al (2008) Understanding the dialysis access steal syndrome. A review of the etiologies, diagnosis, prevention and treatment strategies. J Vasc Access 9 (3):155–166

Muir C, Kotwal S, Hawley C, Polkinghorne K, Gallagher M, Snelling P et al (2014) Buttonhole cannulation and clinical outcomes in a home hemodialysis cohort and systematic review. Clin J Am Soc Nephrol 9 (1):110–119

Norton de Matos A, Sousa C, Teixeira G (2023) Doppler ultrasound in vascular access for haemodialysis. Gráfica de Paredes, Lda, Porto

Padberg FJ, Calligaro K, Sidawy A (2008) Complications of arteriovenous hemodialysis access: recognition and management. J Vasc Surg 48 (5 Suppl):55S–80S

Pasklinsky G, Meisner R, Labropoulos N, Leon L, Gasparis A, Landau D et al (2011) Management of true aneurysms of hemodialysis access fistulas. J Vasc Surg 53 (5):1291–1297

Pinto R, Ferreira E, Sousa C, Barros J, Correia A, Silva A et al (2024) Skin pigmentation as landmark for arteriovenous fistula cannulation in hemodialysis. J Vasc Access 25 (6):1925–1931. https://doi.org/10.1177/11297298231193477

Pinto R, Sousa C, Salgueiro A, Fernandes I (2022) Arteriovenous fistula cannulation in hemodialysis: a vascular access clinical practice guidelines narrative review. J Vasc Access 23 (5):825–831

Quencer K, Arici M (2015) Arteriovenous fistulas and their characteristic sites of stenosis. AJR Am J Roentgenol 205 (4):726–734

Quencer K, Kidd J, Kinney T (2017) Preprocedure evaluation of a dysfunctional dialysis access. Tech Vasc Interv Radiol 20 (1):20–30

Saeed F, Kousar N, Sinnakirouchenan R, Ramalingam VS, Johnson PB, Holley JL (2011) Blood loss through AV fistula: a case report and literature review. Int J Nephrol 2011:350870

Scali S, Huber T (2011) Treatment strategies for access-related hand ischemia. Semin Vasc Surg 24(2):128–136

Scheltinga M, van Hoek F, Bruijninckx C (2009) Time of onset in haemodialysis access-induced distal ischaemia (HAIDI) is related to the access type. Nephrol Dial Transplant 24(10):3198–3204

Schmidli J, Widmer M, Basile C, de Donato G, Gallieni M, Gibbons C et al (2018) Editor's Choice – Vascular Access: 2018 Clinical Practice Guidelines of the European Society for Vascular Surgery (ESVS). Eur J Vasc Endovasc Surg 55(6):757–818

Schneider J, White G, Dejesus E (2012) Pasteurella multocida-infected expanded polytetrafluoroethylene hemodialysis access graft. Ann Vasc Surg 26(8):1128.e15– e17

Siddiky A, Sarwar K, Ahmad N, Gilbert J (2014) Management of arteriovenous fistulas. BMJ 349:g6262

Sousa C, Apóstolo J, Figueiredo M, Martins M, Dias V (2013) Physical examination: how to examine the arm with arteriovenous fistula. Hemodial Int 17(2):300–306

Sousa C, Teles P, Sousa R, Cabrita F, Ribeiro O, Delgado E et al (2024) Hemodialysis vascular access coordinator: three-level model for access management. Semin Dial 37(2):85–90

Stolic R (2013) Most important chronic complications of arteriovenous fistulas for hemodialysis. Med Princ Pract 22(3):220–228

Teixeira G, Almeida P, Loureiro L, Antunes I, Rego D, Teixeira S et al (2021) Arterial percutaneous angioplasty in hemodialysis access: endovascular treatment of hand ischemia. J Vasc Access 22(3):411–416

Teixeira G, Almeida P, Sousa C, Teles P, Sousa P, Loureiro L et al (2017) Arteriovenous access banding revisited. J Vasc Access 18(3):225–231

Tonelli M, Wiebe N, Guthrie B, James M, Quan H, Fortin M et al (2015) Comorbidity as a driver of adverse outcomes in people with chronic kidney disease. Kidney Int 88(4):859–866

Wiese P, Nonnast-Daniel B (2004) Colour Doppler ultrasound in dialysis access. Nephrol Dial Transplant 19(8):1956–1963

Monitoring and Surveillance of an Arteriovenous Fistula

Nurten Ozen and Clemente Neves Sousa

The lifespan of an arteriovenous fistula (AVF) depends on several factors among which an appropriate and continuous monitoring and surveillance have a major importance. The main goals are the detection of problems that may compromise the access or limit its functionality and to seek the best solution for AVF maintenance. This is done in order to enhance the lifespan of the arteriovenous access by decreasing the likelihood of thrombosis (Lok et al. 2020). Identifying and addressing AVF access dysfunction in haemodialysis (HD) early are crucial goals for healthcare providers. This approach aims to decrease complications associated with AVF access, lower hospitalization rates, reduce related costs, and extend the lifespan of AVF access (Salman 2022).

The terms "monitoring" and "surveillance" were introduced and defined by the clinical practice guidelines of the Kidney Disease Outcomes Quality Initiatives. Monitoring involves the use of physical examination along with the identification of clinical and biochemical abnormalities to detect dysfunction in the vascular access. On the other hand, surveillance entails employing specialized equipment to evaluate and pinpoint access dysfunction. The purpose of surveillance tests is to measure the blood flow in the dialysis access (Besarab et al. 2007), either through dynamic or static access venous pressure assessment or by using methods such as the ultrasound dilution technique, or Doppler ultrasonography to assess anatomical irregularities (Thamer et al. 2018; Lok et al. 2020). Vascular access surveillance is recommended

---

N. Ozen (✉)
Faculty of Nursing, Department of Internal Medicine Nursing, Istanbul University, Istanbul, Turkey
e-mail: nurten.ozen@istanbul.edu.tr

C. N. Sousa
Nursing School of University of Porto, Porto, Portugal
e-mail: clementesousa@esenf.pt

RISE – Health, University of Porto, Porto, Portugal

© The Author(s), under exclusive license to Springer Nature Switzerland AG 2025
N. Ozen et al. (eds.), *Arteriovenous Fistula Management*,
https://doi.org/10.1007/978-3-032-04771-7_5

to be carried out through flow measurements in the AVF every 3 months (Schmidli et al. 2018) or when changes of the access functionality occur that need to be analyzed. However, the monitoring and surveillance program should be adjusted to the access characteristics and tailored to each individual patient.

Monitoring is the primary method used for early detection of AVF access problems. AVF access monitoring involves physical examination of clinical indicators of AVF dysfunction, such as extended bleeding, edema in the extremities on the same side as the AVF access, high recirculation rates, inappropriate dialysis, frequent dialysis machine alarms, cannulation difficulties, and formation of aneurysms, among other problems (Sousa et al. 2013, 2023; Thamer et al. 2018). Routine physical examination is recommended for monitoring and maintenance of the vascular access by trained professionals (Sousa et al. 2014). The importance and advantages of consistently monitoring the HD access are widely acknowledged (Lok et al. 2020). It is recommended that monitoring should take place at a minimum frequency of once a month. Furthermore, the guidelines from the 2019 Kidney Disease Outcomes Quality Initiative (KDOQI) state that there is insufficient evidence to suggest the use of regular AVF surveillance, along with routine standard clinical monitoring, to enhance the patency of AVF access (Lok et al. 2020).

Vascular access surveillance refers to the systematic use of tools and instruments for conducting regular, periodic assessments of the HD vascular access, aimed at early detection of stenotic lesions (Lok et al. 2020). The available evidence is insufficient for KDOQI to formulate a recommendation regarding routine AVF surveillance. While numerous surveillance methods have been developed to identify vascular stenosis (Lok et al. 2020), three primary approaches have traditionally been employed. This includes measurements of access blood flow, pressure monitoring, or imaging for detecting stenosis. Such surveillance would be supplementary to regular clinical monitoring, with the aim of enhancing access patency.

Surveillance methods, which require specialized equipment and operator expertise, have been researched for their ability to identify stenosis prior to the emergence of clinical signs. These methods encompass measuring arteriovenous access flow (Q_a) using several techniques, such as ultrasound dilution method and duplex ultrasound, which measure Q_a and provide visualization of anatomical irregularities. Additionally, the static venous pressure has been employed as surveillance tools, although dynamic venous pressure measurements are now regarded as complementary to clinical monitoring (Fig. 1) (Lok et al. 2020).

The theoretical objectives of AVF follow-up programs encompass several key goals, including early detection of AVF stenosis, reduction of AVF thrombosis rate, improvement in AVF patency, enhanced frequency of planned AVF interventions, decrease the need for emergency AVF interventions and for the creation of new AVFs, lower incidence of hospitalizations related to AVF complications, fewer missed HD sessions, reduction in the need for catheter placement, and decrease in overall healthcare costs (Wijnen et al. 2006).

In other words, the primary focus is on vascular access monitoring, while the findings from surveillance serve as supplementary information. Decisions and actions should not solely rely on the surveillance results (Lok et al. 2020). Monitoring and surveillance can be divided into first-generation methods (physical examination, access pressure, recirculation, and unexplained drop in dialysis adequacy) and

Methods of Monitoring and Surveillance			
	Physical Examination	Monitoring[1]	First-generation methods[2]
	Pressure of Arteriovenous Fistula		
	Evaluation of Recirculation		
	Unexplained Drop in Dialysis Adequacy		
	Doppler Ultrasound	Surveillance[1]	Second-generation methods[2]
	Dilution Screening Methods		

1 – KDOQI Clinical Practice Guideline for Vascular Access: 2019 Update
2 – Spanish Clinical Guidelines on Vascular Access for Haemodialysis

Fig. 1 AVF monitoring and surveillance methods

second-generation methods (which enable calculation of the access flow), according to the Spanish guidelines (Ibeas et al. 2017). The fundamental principle of vascular access monitoring and surveillance is to detect faulty access points, enable timely intervention, and ultimately reduce interruptions of the dialysis treatment.

1 Monitoring of the Arteriovenous Fistula

AVF monitoring is a fundamental component in the management of the arteriovenous access in HD patients, enabling early problem detection. This process is based on integrating the clinical method (physical examination) with the data/information resulting from the analysis of the AVF (pressures, recirculation, cannulation problems, and hemostasis) with the aim of improving the patency and efficiency of the vascular access (Sousa et al. 2013; Ibeas et al. 2017).

The implementation of continuous monitoring strategies is key for maintaining the functionality of the AVF, reducing the incidence of complications and the need for urgent intervention. Furthermore, early detection of abnormalities enables the adoption of preventive therapeutic measures, improving clinical results.

Physical Examination

The physical examination must be conducted carefully and is always the initial step used to diagnose and treat a malfunctioning access. A combined approach of physical examination and the data/information resulting from AVF analysis should be considered rather than relying solely on technological results (Koirala et al. 2016). According to the KDOQI guidelines, the AVF should be physically examined before each cannulation (Lok et al. 2020). Physical examination (summary and systematic) of an AVF was discussed in Chap. 3.

In addition to the findings obtained from physical examination, the physical characteristics of the access while the patient is on dialysis can provide hints of complications such as direct signs of distal perfusion changes in the hand or indirect signs of AVF stenosis if they appear persistently (three consecutive HD sessions) compared to previous HD sessions. These signs may include difficulties in AVF needling and/or cannulation (Sousa et al. 2023), aspiration of clots during needling, increase in negative pre-pump arterial pressure, failure to reach prescribed blood flow rate (Q_b), increase in the return or venous pressure, and prolonged hemostasis time, without excessive anticoagulation. Prolonged bleeding (>20 minutes) from the needle sites after HD is complete might indicate an underlying outflow stenosis, as the flow tends to follow the path of least resistance. However, prolonged bleeding is not specific to stenosis, as underlying coagulopathy or the use of therapeutic anticoagulants may also contribute to the situation. Recurrent clotting (occurring at least twice per month) could be another indicator (Ibeas et al. 2017; Whittier 2009; UpToDate 2023).

Pressures of Arteriovenous Fistula

The assessment should also be carried out during the first 1.5 hours of treatment in order to eliminate errors caused by a decrease in cardiac output or blood pressure related to ultrafiltration or hypotension (Salman 2022). Flow monitoring is the optimal surveillance method for AVF stenosis, most likely due to the fact that an AVF is a low-pressure system. Intra-access blood flow can be measured using a number of methods. Published literature indicates that all methods of flow monitoring generally provide similar values. Dialysis access blood flow measurements are typically conducted on a monthly basis (Bodington et al. 2020; UpToDate 2023). The presence of a stenosis leads to a decrease in the venous outflow, accompanied by a simultaneous increase in the pressure in the arterial inflow (Koirala et al. 2016).

Arterial pre-pump blood pressure is essential to assess the AVF function and the effectiveness of HD treatment. Abnormal pressures, whether low or high, reflect problems with the AVF. Extremely negative blood pressure (< -300 mmHg, with $Qb = 300$ ml/min) show blood flow problems, consistent with inflow problems (Sousa 2012). Slightly negative blood pressure (> -150 mmHg, with $Qb = 300$ ml/min) may also indicate inflow problems associated with recirculation (Sousa 2012). Such situations lead to a reduction in the volume of dialyzed blood and the effectiveness of dialysis. Changes in this pressure may indicate inflow problems such as stenosis and increase the risk of thrombosis.

Direct venous pressure (DVP) measurement and static pressure measurement are the two pressure parameters employed in flow calculations (Ibeas et al. 2017; Whitter 2009; Koirala et al. 2016; UpToDate 2023). DVP is measured when extracorporeal blood is present. DVP can be measured at the start of dialysis because it requires low blood flow rates (50–225 ml/min) and employs 15-gauge needles to gauge blood flow (Koirala et al. 2016; UpToDate 2023). However, this approach does not yield consistently reliable results, as the use of differently sized needles can affect the pressure value as well as the prescribed blood flow. With higher blood flow rates, if needle sizes are not adjusted, it is harder for blood to pass through the needles and resistance increases with rising venous pressure. In this situation, the increase in venous pressure is due to needle size and not to access problems. These issues make measurement less reliable.

KDOQI guidelines warn against using unstandardized DVP as an indicator for outflow stenosis (Koirala et al. 2016; Ibeas et al. 2017). Static venous pressure refers to the pressure within the access when extracorporeal blood flow is absent or before the start of HD. This method is more dependable than DVP because it involves fewer variables (Whittier 2009; Bodington et al. 2020). It does not require the variables associated with DVP such as needle size, machine type, and blood flow, making it a more reliable measurement. This method is adjusted for variations in height between the venous needle in the access and the venous drip chamber, and it is also normalized for the mean arterial pressure (MAP). The normalized ratio of intra-access pressure (IAP) at the arterial and venous end to the MAP is computed as follows: Arterial ratio = (arterial IAP + arterial height correction) / MAP. Venous ratio = (venous IAP + venous height correction) / MAP (Koirala et al. 2016). Intra-access pressure measurement methods encompass both direct and indirect approaches. Direct methods involve pressure measurement using a pressure-measuring device at the cannulation sites. Indirectly, intra-access pressure can be assessed using the HD machine itself which is based on the pressures from the arterial pre-pump and "venous" post-pump drip chambers when the blood pump is deactivated (Sharma and Ranjan 2014).

Evaluation of Recirculation

Access recirculation refers to the situation where dialyzed blood is immediately directed back to the dialysis machine instead of re-entering the patient's circulatory system. Turbulent and nonlinear flow, along with recirculation, typically indicates the existence of a stenosis upstream of the access point. This recirculation contributes to dialysis inefficiency and usually serves as a sign of an abnormality within the access. Recirculation can also arise from incorrect placement of bloodline needles or insufficient spacing between needles, leading to the possibility of false positive results (Koirala et al. 2016). Therefore, the measurement of recirculation is not the best method for early detection of stenosis (Tonelli et al. 2001). Furthermore, it is worth noting that the presence of a localized stenosis between the two AVF needles does not result in recirculation (Whittier 2009). Venous stenosis stands out as one of the most prevalent factors behind recirculation because the blood that re-enters the venous limb has trouble exiting the access, causing the same blood to be subjected to another round of dialysis. Access recirculation is gauged using methods based on urea, blood temperature monitoring, or indicator dilution techniques (Koirala et al. 2016).

AVF recirculation is composed of two distinct components: vascular access recirculation and cardiopulmonary recirculation. The former transpires when blood returning to the access is drawn back into the arterial line, bypassing the patient, due to the blood pump's rate exceeding Q_a. This situation hampers effective dialysis by preventing equalization of dialyzed and non-dialyzed blood. Numerous factors contribute to vascular access recirculation, encompassing access flow, pump speed, positioning and distance of needle tips, line orientation, access stenosis, and type. Conversely, cardiopulmonary recirculation involves dialyzed blood being redirected back to the vascular access and ultimately the heart via the venous system, without adequately reaching the peripheral tissues. In cases of patients with cardiac ailments or compromised perfusion, the peripheral circulation is suboptimal, hindering the proper balance of dialyzed blood with poorly perfused tissue. Cardiopulmonary recirculation frequently goes unnoticed for extended periods, often due to insufficient attention, and it can be significant in certain patients (Fedderson and Roger 2012).

Recirculation has traditionally been assessed using urea-based techniques. However, alternative methods that do not rely on urea have also been proposed. These include ultrasound dilution, potassium dilution, ionic dialysance, glucose infusion, and thermal dilution methods (Whittier 2009). Arteriovenous access recirculation and declines in the urea reduction rate (URR) or Kt/V may help indicate arteriovenous access stenosis, but they alone cannot be sole indicators because many variables affect their measurements and they have not been rigorously studied (Lok et al. 2020).

Unexplained Drop in Dialysis Adequacy

The Kt/V measurement has been proposed as an objective assessment technique for an AVF (Schmidli et al. 2018). Nonetheless, it is influenced by a number of factors beyond just urea clearance, such as the duration of HD and the Q_b, both of which can impact Kt/V values. Therefore, it is essential to incorporate the recirculation rate as a parameter in the functional evaluation of an AVF. However, many other factors influence Kt/V and URR, making them less sensitive and less specific for detecting vascular access dysfunction (Schmidli et al. 2018).

2 Surveillance of the Arteriovenous Fistula

A number of techniques have been used to measure access flow including duplex ultrasound. Ultrasound flow dilution, glucose pump test, and ionic dialysance also have been used to determine Q_a. At present, no technique has been conclusively proven to improve outcomes in the management of complications related to access thrombosis. Moreover, the ideal frequency to monitor access flow has not been determined. The technique used to measure Q_a should be easy to use in a routine clinical setting with little interoperator variability and high sensitivity and specificity (Fluck and Kumwenda 2011; Ibeas et al. 2017). The best method of measuring access blood flow should be readily available as a routine screening tool.

Doppler Ultrasound

The doppler ultrasound (DUS) is the main imaging modality for vascular access surveillance. DUS can enhance the understanding of the physiology and pathology of every vascular access (Schmidli et al. 2018). DUS examination offers prompt and valuable insights into various aspects, including studying the wall and diameters of vascular structures, evaluating the diameter of surgical anastomoses, identifying the presence of haematoma, fibrosis, edema, vascular calcifications, aneurysms, and pseudoaneurysms, detecting morphological stenosis or veins with reduced size, visualizing collateral veins, assessing vessel tortuosity, determining the proximity of the efferent vein to the afferent artery, and identifying the presence of partial or total AVF thrombosis (Ibeas et al. 2017). In a meta-analysis conducted by Ali et al. (2021), the authors recommend conducting regular HD access surveillance using noninvasive ultrasound techniques to lower the risk of vascular access thrombosis in patients with AVF.

Dilution Screening Method

These techniques are grounded in Fick's principle. In the course of dialysis, a saline solution is introduced into the dialysis tubing, and either an ultrasound or heat/light sensor is used to monitor the dilution of blood within the dialysis lines. These data are then employed to compute the rates of access flow. The methodology involves interchanging the positions of the lines' arterial and venous segments and ensuring the arterial line is downstream from the venous return line. Consequently, the blood that has been dialyzed and is being returned into the access is collected (recirculated) by the arterial line, which directs the blood into the dialyzer. Flow dilution sensors are clamped onto both the arterial and venous segments. A bolus of saline is introduced into the venous line, and the dilution sensor gauges the extent of dilution. This diluted blood traverses the access, and a portion of this diluted blood is drawn into the arterial segment through the action of the blood pump (Ahmad 2017).

According to the European guidelines, there is no distinct preference for any specific method among these techniques (Tordoir et al. 2007). Most studies have indicated comparable results for Q_a when different dilution techniques are applied. Indeed, each method has its own advantages and disadvantages. For instance, thermodilution and temperature gradient have an edge over the aforementioned techniques because the sensor is already integrated into the HD machine. However, the Q_a value is not automatically recorded and needs subsequent computation. Both methods are solely validated for high-flux HD with Q_b of 300 ml/min. The use of certain devices enables the instant inversion of the HD blood lines, considerably reducing the time required to find the Q_a value (Ibeas et al. 2017). Ibeas et al. (2017) recommend using both Doppler ultrasound and dilution screening methods interchangeably in order to assess the AVF function. These methods exhibit equivalent performance for blood flow determination. The dilution techniques that require reversing the blood lines in HD are the ones predominantly employed nowadays. Nonetheless, certain scenarios preclude their application. For instance, when the venous needle, responsible for blood return, is inserted into a vein other than the arterialized vein connected to the AVF, recirculation of blood within the AVF is nil. Consequently, determining Q_a becomes unfeasible (Wijinen et al. 2007; Tiranathanagul et al. 2008). Dilution methods employed to calculate Q_a during HD should be conducted within the initial hour of the session. This timing is essential to prevent hemodynamic fluctuations arising as a result of ultrafiltration (Ibeas et al. 2017).

Ultrasound Dilution Method

The use of the ultrasound dilution technique (UDT) is somewhat restricted due to the following reasons: the measurement requires specialized instruments; the procedure must be conducted during the dialysis session; both the arterial and venous lines need to be inserted into the same vein; and reversing the blood lines is essential, which is both inconvenient and time-consuming (Steuer et al. 2001). This was the first dilution method described. An external monitor, a Doppler sensor placed on each HD line, and an isotonic saline bolus (indicator) administered for 6–8 seconds into the arterial line are used both in the normal position and after the blood lines are reversed during hemodialysis (Ibeas et al. 2017).

Hematocrit Dilution Method or Delta-H

In order to overcome the UDT limitations, a new and straightforward method for measuring Q_a has been developed. This innovative approach is grounded on the dilution principle of red blood cell concentration. This method, known as the hemoglobin dilution technique (HDT), circumvents the need for specialized instruments and employs only standard HD equipment and materials. In the HDT, the determination of Q_a involves reversing the HD circuit, similar to the UDT. In the HDT, the process is streamlined. Only two samples of either haemoglobin or hematocrit are required: one taken as a baseline before commencing the HD session, and the other collected 12 seconds after initiating the blood pump for the priming saline infusion, with the circuit reversed. These samples are then used to calculate Q_a (Tiranathanagul et al. 2008).

Thermodilution Method

The thermodilution technique relies on the occurrence of changes of the dialysate temperature upon its amalgamation with blood, facilitating the computation of the intra-access blood flow rate. Temperature-sensitive thermistors are positioned within the arterial and venous lines. Such thermistors detect temperature changes downstream over a specific time frame as a cold injectate is introduced into the access. A blood temperature monitor gauges temperature changes, enabling computation of the flow rate based on the mean blood temperature and the duration of the injectate's transit (Schneditz et al. 1998).

Temperature Gradient Method

The temperature gradient method was introduced and validated by Wijnen et al. (2007) through a comparison with the ultrasound dilution method. Q_a can be checked by using the Blood Temperature Monitoring sensor integrated into certain HD machines. The temperature gradient technique enables calculation of Q_a by analyzing temperature values acquired from HD lines positioned normally and then reversed, sparing the requirement to make a temperature bolus (Ibeas et al. 2017).

Ionic Dialysance Method

Recent progress has enabled real-time online measurement of the "effective ionic dialysance" (EID), serving as an indicator of the delivered dialysis dose (Lindsay et al. 2001). EID can replace the effective urea clearance because the diffusivity of NaCl closely approaches that of urea across the dialyzer membrane. Additionally, the sodium osmotic distribution volume matches the volume of urea distribution which is equivalent to the total body water (Gotch et al. 2004). The effectiveness of ionic dialysance also depends on the Q_b and dialysate flow rates, particularly during high-flux HD. Although efforts have been made to employ EID for evaluating access flow, such attempts have run into limitations in terms of practical application (Ibeas et al. 2017).

3 Vascular Access Management Models

Several studies have shown that having a vascular access management program in place increases the number of AVFs, reduces central venous catheters, and reduces patient hospitalizations related to the vascular access. Implementation of monitoring and surveillance programs is essential to promote treatment effectiveness and reduces both morbidity and mortality (van Loon et al. 2007; Pundir et al. 2022; Sousa et al. 2024).

The available literature shows how to organize vascular access management, combining vascular access monitoring and surveillance. According to such management models, it is important to offer education and training to the entire team, with the aim of developing skills to detect AVF dysfunction and clarifying the role of each team member.

The three-level model (3Level_M) is a vascular access management model based on a hierarchy composed of three essential functions, each with a specific role in monitoring/surveillance, intervention, and coordination of the vascular access (Sousa et al. 2024). The first level is the nurse responsible for the vascular access, whose main responsibility is to carry out the systematic physical examination, analyze the recommendations for cannulation (Sousa et al. 2023), implement monitoring and/or surveillance programs, and train the patient. The nurse must have specific training on vascular access and it must be carried out in a clinical setting using simulation (Sousa et al. 2024).

The second level is the coordinator, who plays a key role in vascular access management. This professional is responsible for the early detection of dysfunction, defining the action plan, coordinating appropriate intervention, and educating/training the entire dialysis team. In addition, the coordinator is the link between the nursing team, the nephrologist and vascular surgeon, and other professionals, ensuring effective communication and an integrated approach to patient care (Sousa et al. 2024).

The third level is the vascular access consultant with extensive experience and in-depth knowledge of the area, who advises and supports the coordinator. This expert promotes counselling and the discussion/reflection process, enabling the coordinator to develop their decision-making skills (Sousa et al. 2024). In addition, 3Level_M improves communication between the professionals involved and guarantees more qualified and safer care for HD patients (Sousa et al. 2024).

Vascular access management models promote a more efficient and organized approach, enhancing early problem detection, reducing urgent interventions, and increasing the patency of vascular accesses.

4 Practical Implications

Access monitoring and surveillance involve an interdisciplinary team collaboration. The team should include the patient, the nephrologist, the nephrology nurse, the technician, the interventional radiologist/nephrologist, the surgeon, and the primary care physician. Additionally, social workers and dietitians can also contribute to this ongoing effort. Physical examination and clinical assessment play a crucial role in access maintenance and should be integral to the standard care of dialysis patients. Q_a and venous pressure measurements can serve as supplementary tests to validate clinical suspicions of stenosis or access dysfunction. The objective should be to accurately identify accesses that are highly likely to benefit from pre-emptive intervention, while refraining from performing procedures on accesses with lower likelihood of improvement. Each dialysis facility should implement a regular Access Monitoring/Surveillance Program. This program aims to detect and address vascular access issues, improve the long-term function of access points, and decrease the expenses linked with maintaining access patency. Education and training, encompassing all professionals engaged in the process, are a pivotal component for establishing a viable monitoring program. This comprehensive training should cover aspects such as an in-depth understanding of vascular access anatomy, its functional dynamics, and clinical assessment techniques.

References

Ahmad S (2017) Outpatient surveillance at the dialysis center. In: Shalhub S, Dua A, Shin S (eds.). Hemodialysis access: fundamentals and advanced management. Springer International Publishing, Switzerland, 173–182

Ali H, Mohamed MM, Baharani J (2021) Effects of hemodialysis access surveillance on reducing risk of hemodialysis access thrombosis: a meta-analysis of randomized studies. Hemodial Int https://doi.org/10.1111/hdi.12927

Besarab A, Asif A, Roy-Chaudhury P, Spergel LM, Ravani P (2007) The native arteriovenous fistula in 2007 Surveillance and monitoring. J Nephrol 20(6):656–667. PMID: 18046667

Bodington R, Greenley S, Bhandari S (2020) Getting the basics right: the monitoring of arteriovenous fistulae, a review of the evidence. Curr Opin Nephrol Hypertens 29(6):564–571. https://doi.org/10.1097/MNH.0000000000000644

Feddersen MA, Roger SD (2012) Arteriovenous fistula surveillance: everyone's responsibility. Port J Nephrol Hypert 26(4):255–265

Fluck R, Kumwenda M (2011) Renal Association Clinical Practice Guideline on vascular access for haemodialysis. Nephron Clin Pract 118(Suppl 1):c225–c240. https://doi.org/10.1159/000328071

Gotch FA, Panlilio FM, Buyaki RA, Wang EX, Folden TI, Levin NW (2004) Mechanisms determining the ratio of conductivity clearance to urea clearance. Kidney Int 66(Suppl 89):S3–S24. https://doi.org/10.1111/j.1523-1755.2004.00759.x

Ibeas J, Roca-Tey R, Vallespín J, Moreno T, Moñux G, Martí-Monrós A et al (2017) Spanish Clinical Guidelines on Vascular Access for Haemodialysis. Nefrologia 37(Suppl 1):1–191. https://doi.org/10.1016/j.nefro.2017.11.004

Koirala N, Anvari E, McLennan G (2016) Monitoring and surveillance of hemodialysis access. Semin Intervent Radiol 33(1):25–30. https://doi.org/10.1055/s-0036-1572548

Lindsay RM, Bene B, Goux N, Heidenheim AP, Landgren C, Sternby J (2001) Relationship between effective ionic dialysance and in vivo urea clearance during hemodialysis. Am J Kidney Dis 38(3):565–574. https://doi.org/10.1053/ajkd.2001.26874

Lok CE, Huber TS, Lee T, Shenoy S, Yevzlin AS, Abreo K et al (2020) KDOQI Clinical Practice Guideline for Vascular Access: 2019 update. Am J Kidney Dis 75(4 Suppl 2):S1–S164. https://doi.org/10.1053/j.ajkd.2019.12.001

Pundir E, Sharma A, Singh S, Patil S, Pandey G, Rally S et al (2022) Impact of a trained vascular access coordinator on a vascular access program in India. J Vasc Access 23(4):495–499

Salman L (2022) Approach to an abnormal surveillance measurement. In: Yevzlin AS, Asif A, Salman L, Ramani K, Qaqish SS, Vacharajani TJ (eds.). Interventional nephrology: principles and practices, 2nd edn, Springer, Switzerland, pp 159–163

Schneditz D, Fan Z, Kaufman A, Levin NW (1998) Measurement of access flow during hemodialysis using the constant infusion approach. ASAIO J 44(1):74–81. https://doi.org/10.1097/00002480-199801000-00015

Schmidli J, Widmer MK, Basile C et al (2018) Vascular access: 2018 clinical practice guidelines of the European Society for Vascular Surgery (ESVS). Eur J Vasc Endovasc Surg 55:757–818

Sharma A, Ranjan P (2014) Arteriovenous fistula (AVF) monitoring and surveillance. Clin Queries Nephrol. 3(1):46–50

Sousa C (2012) Caring for the person arteriovenous fistula: model for continuous improvement. Rev Port Sau Pub 30(1):11–17

Sousa C, Apóstolo J, Figueiredo M, Martins M, Dias V (2013) Physical examination: how to examine the arm with arteriovenous fistula. Hemodial Int 17(2):300–306

Sousa C, Teles P, Dias V, Apóstolo J, Figueiredo M, Martins M (2014) Physical examination of arteriovenous fistula: the influence of professional experience in the detection of complications. Hemodial Int 18(3):695–699

Sousa C, Teles P, Ribeiro O, Sousa R, Lira M, Delgado E et al (2023) How to choose the appropriate cannulation technique for vascular access in hemodialysis patients. Ther Apher Dial 27(3):394–401

Sousa C, Teles P, Sousa R, Cabrita F, Ribeiro O, Delgado E et al (2024) Hemodialysis vascular access coordinator: three-level model for access management. Semin Dial 37(2):85–90

Steuer RR, Miller DR, Zhang S, Bell DA, Leypoldt JK (2001) Noninvasive transcutaneous determination of access blood flow rate. Kidney Int 60(1):284–291. https://doi.org/10.1046/j.1523-1755.2001.00798.x

Thamer M, Lee TC, Wasse H, Glickman MH, Qian J, Gottlieb D et al (2018) Medicare costs associated with arteriovenous fistulas among US hemodialysis patients. Am J Kidney Dis 72(1):10–18. https://doi.org/10.1053/j.ajkd.2018.01.034

Tiranathanagul K, Katavetin P, Injan P, Leelahavanichkul A, Techawathanawanna N, Praditpornsilpa K et al (2008) A novel simple hemoglobin dilution technique to measure hemodialysis vascular access flow. Kidney Int 73(9):1082–1086. https://doi.org/10.1038/ki.2008.10

Tonelli M, Jindal K, Hirsch D, Taylor S, Kane C, Henbrey S (2001) Screening for subclinical stenosis in native vessel arteriovenous fistulae. J Am Soc Nephrol 12(8):1729–1733. https://doi.org/10.1681/ASN.V1281729

Tordoir J, Canaud B, Haage P, Konner K, Basci A, Fouque D et al (2007) EBPG on vascular access. Nephrol Dial Transplant 22(Suppl 2):ii88–117. https://doi.org/10.1093/ndt/gfm021

UpToDate (2023) Clinical monitoring and surveillance of the mature hemodialysis arteriovenous fistula. https://www.uptodate.com/contents/clinical-monitoring-and-surveillance-of-the-mature-hemodialysis-arteriovenous-fistula?search=Clinical%20monitoring%20and%20surveillance%20of%20hemodialysis%20arteriovenous%20fistula&source=search_result&selectedTitle=1~150&usage_type=default&display_rank=1#H606471974. Accessed 23 Aug 2023

van Loon M, van der Mark W, Beukers N, Bruin C, Blankestijn P, Huisman R et al (2007) Implementation of a vascular access quality programme improves vascular access care. Nephrol Dial Transplant 22(6):1628–1632

Whittier WL (2009) Surveillance of hemodialysis vascular access. Semin Intervent Radiol 26:130–138. https://doi.org/10.1055/s-0029-1222457

Wijnen E, Planken N, Keuter X, Kooman JP, Tordoir JH, De Haan MW et al (2006) Impact of a quality improvement programme based on vascular access flow monitoring on costs, access occlusion and access failure. Nephrol Dial Transplant 21:3514–3519

Wijnen E, van der Sande FM, Kooman JP, de Graaf T, Tordoir JH, Leunissen KM et al (2007) Measurement of hemodialysis vascular access flow using extracorporeal temperature gradients. Kidney Int 72(6):736–741. https://doi.org/10.1038/sj.ki.5002376

Cannulation Methods for the Arteriovenous Fistula

Clemente Neves Sousa, Nurten Ozen, and Paulo Teles

The arteriovenous fistula (AVF) is considered by the scientific community as the best vascular access for haemodialysis patients. Quality and patency of the AVF do not depend solely on the vascular network, the surgeon's experience, monitoring and surveillance programmes, or self-care behaviours performed by patients, but also on cannulation. However, the selected cannulation method may influence both patency and the rate of complications associated with an AVF, namely the type of cannulation technique used, the needle-type selection, the cannulation site, cannulation preparation, and the ratio patient/nurse (Sousa et al. 2023).

C. N. Sousa (✉)
Nursing School of University of Porto, Porto, Portugal
e-mail: clementesousa@esenf.pt

RISE – Health, University of Porto, Porto, Portugal

N. Ozen
Faculty of Nursing, Department of Internal Medicine Nursing, Istanbul University, Istanbul, Turkey
e-mail: nurten.ozen@istanbul.edu.tr

P. Teles
School of Economics, University of Porto, Porto, Portugal
e-mail: pteles@fep.up.pt

LIAAD-INESC Porto LA, Porto, Portugal

© The Author(s), under exclusive license to Springer Nature Switzerland AG 2025
N. Ozen et al. (eds.), *Arteriovenous Fistula Management*,
https://doi.org/10.1007/978-3-032-04771-7_6

1 Cannulation Method

Arteriovenous-fistula cannulation is a complex process that should not be limited to the needling or cannulation technique. The cannulation method involves aspects of pre-cannulation (identification of the access flow, selection of the cannulation site and type of needle, and preparation for cannulation), cannulation (cannulation technique and needle bevel position), and post-cannulation (needle removal and haemostasis process) (Sousa 2012; Pinto et al. 2022). During the cannulation, the nurse also employs ultrasound as an adjunct to refine clinical judgment and optimize cannulation-related decisions. Such aspects allow the cannulation method to be tailored so that the nephrologist nurse can prescribe each patient the appropriate cannulation technique.

Pre-cannulation

At this point, identifying the type of arteriovenous access and the flow direction is key. Physical examination must be carried out before cannulation with the aim of assisting in the recognition and identification of the venous network (especially the draining vein) in order to examine the thrill and detect the presence of thrombosis/problem segments in the draining vein (Sousa et al. 2013, 2023).

Identification of the AVF flow enables finding the appropriate location for cannulation and designing a strategy to preserve the venous network. Site selection should be made in the same segment of the fistula as often as possible. If the patient has a distal AVF, cannulations will preferably be in the forearm (Sousa 2012; Pinto et al. 2022). However, in some situations, it may be advisable to cannulate the arm, depending on the location of the AVF. In addition to physical examination, the use of ultrasound offers a complementary and highly valuable assessment of AVF. Ultrasound allows for the evaluation of the morphology vascular and structure vascular of the AVF, enables direct visualisation of vascular anatomy, confirmation of flow direction, an identification of the endothelial problems, aneurysms or thrombus, Chap. 8.

Arterial cannulation can be antegrade (in the direction of the flow) or retrograde (against the flow) at a distance of 2–3 cm from the anastomosis (Sousa 2009; Sousa et al. 2023), whereas venous cannulation is always made in the direction of the flow, in an antegrade position, and 5 cm away from arterial cannulation, that is, 7–8 cm from anastomosis (Sousa et al. 2023). A systematic and meta-analysis study with 249 haemodialysis (HD) patients showed that when needles are placed less than 5 cm apart, the Kt/V and access recirculation are greater than when placed more than 5 cm apart (Karkhah et al. 2023). Concerning the direction of the needle, this study does not find significant differences in the effect of Kt/V or access recirculation, regardless of whether it is antegrade or retrograde (Karkhah et al. 2023).

The nephrologist nurse must promote the use of needles with a diameter appropriate to the venous network, arterial pressure, and prescribed blood flow, with the aim of improving mortality and morbidity without additional costs. Needle diameter can range from 17G (smallest diameter) to 14G (largest diameter). The 16G and 15G needles allow a blood flow of 250–350 ml/min and 300–450 ml/min, respectively (Dinwiddie et al. 2013). Monitoring pre-pump blood pressure can help determine whether the needle diameter should be increased. If arterial pressure is lower than −200/−250 mmHg, the needle should be switched to another with a lower diameter. If blood pressure is lower than −200/−250 mmHg, the needle must be switched to another with a lower-gauge needle (Brouwer 2011; Dinwiddie et al. 2013). Meanwhile, the use of 14G needles in venous cannulation induces no significant improvement in KT/V, no increase of pain or haemostasis time (Mehta et al. 2002; Mondueri et al. 2006). The back-eye needle should be used for the arterial cannulation in order to optimize blood flow and avoid needle manipulation and trauma to the vessel wall.

Cannulation preparation is not just the disinfection process associated with skin cleansing (Pinto et al. 2022). This process should begin with a policy put in practice by the dialysis unit of washing the AVF arm prior to cannulation (Sousa et al. 2023). Patients should be taught and trained to wash their arm before haemodialysis treatment. Washing the AVF arm should be an integral part of AVF care and not optional. Skin disinfection is important to reduce microorganisms that cause infection. Using antimicrobial solutions can reduce this risk. There are many solutions that can be used, with different action times, as well as different application ways. More important than the solution used is respecting the action way and times of each solution to obtain the desired disinfectant effect (Sousa et al. 2023).

Cannulation

The selection of the appropriate AVF cannulation technique is vital for the success of HD. An HD patient needs more than 300 cannulations per year to complete the treatment (van Loon et al. 2009). There are three cannulation techniques described in the literature for haemodialysis patients with AVF: area cannulation, buttonhole cannulation, and roper-ladder cannulation (Sousa et al. 2023).

Concerning the area cannulation technique, cannulations (arterial and venous) are always located in the same area, with a diameter of 2–3 cm. Systematic cannulations in the same location destroy the elastic properties of the vein, enhancing the development of aneurysms and post-aneurysmal stenosis (Sousa et al. 2023). With this type of technique, patients feel less pain during cannulation and nurses report that cannulation is easier when such aneurysms occur.

The buttonhole cannulation technique is described by Twardowski and Kubara, 1979, (Twardowski 2015). This technique is used in Europe and Japan and is well accepted by patients undergoing home haemodialysis and self-cannulation. It must comply with the principles defined by the authors. The same nephrologist nurse or patient must select the cannulation sites (arterial and venous) and perform cannulation with sharp needles in exactly the same orifice and at the same angle during 9–12 HD sessions (Twardowski 2015). During this time, a cylindrical scar tissue develops along the puncture path which leads to the formation of a subcutaneous tunnel from the skin to the vein (Nesrallah 2016; Sousa et al. 2023). After the tunnel is formed, the needle slides through the tunnel into the vein using blunt needles. With such a technique, patients feel less pain during cannulation and nurses report fewer haematomas, aneurysms, and shorter haemostasis time (Bushey 2020).

Regarding the roper-ladder cannulation technique, cannulations (arterial and venous) are systematically distributed along the entire length of the drainage vein, with a defined distance (Pinto et al. 2022). The steps and aspects to be considered in order to implement this technique are described and defined in Sousa et al. (2023). In the first step, the nurse must determine with ultrasound, if possible, the length of the drainage vein that can be cannulated. In the second step, the cannulated drainage vein is split into two segments (which will correspond to the arterial and venous segments). In the third step, the nurse defines the cannulation sites, considering a distance of 2 cm between each cannulation. In the arterial part, the cannulation site A1 (0 cm) is determined first, followed by A2 (2 cm) and A3 (4 cm), corresponding to a distance of 4 cm (0 cm–2 cm–4 cm). After identifying A3, the nurse returns to the beginning but starts 1 cm above A1. This is cannulation site A4 and is followed by A5 (3 cm) and A3 (5 cm), corresponding to a distance of 4 cm (1 cm–3 cm–5 cm) (Fig. 1) (Sousa et al. 2023). Concerning the venous segment, the same process must be carried out in order to determine the cannulation sites, with each one representing a step. Thus, implementing such a technique requires three locations in the arterial and venous parts (Sousa et al. 2023). Then, patients report more pain during cannulation and nurses report more hematomas, fewer aneurysms, and uniform vein drainage with this type of technique.

Literature shows the position of the needle bevel can influence pain and bleeding time after removing the needles. Several studies have shown a statistically significant pain reduction in the bevel down position of antegrade needle insertion compared to the bevel up needle position (Crespo 1994; Crespo Montero et al. 2004; Akyol Durmaz et al. 2015; Ozen et al. 2022). Regarding the incidence of bleeding after needle removal, bleeding occurred more frequently when cannulation was carried out with the bevel up than with it down, which has been shown by proportions of 6.9% and 0.26% respectively (Gaspar et al. 2003). In another study, bleeding time was better when the bevel was down than when it was up (4.76 minutes vs 5.89 minutes, $p < 0.001$) and needles were in the anterograde position (Ozen et al. 2022).

The position of the needle bevel must be adjusted according to the direction of blood flow: in antegrade insertion, the bevel is downwards and in retrograde insertion the bevel is upwards.

Post-cannulation

The process of needle removal is just as important as inserting them. This process must be careful in order to avoid/prevent trauma to the vein and post-dialysis haematomas/infiltrations.

The needles should be removed after the blood has returned to the extracorporeal circuit, measuring blood pressure and ensuring the patient is in a position to perform haemostasis. Needles must be withdrawn at the same angle as they were inserted to avoid the bevel "dragging" on the vessel and skin (Sousa 2009). During the process,

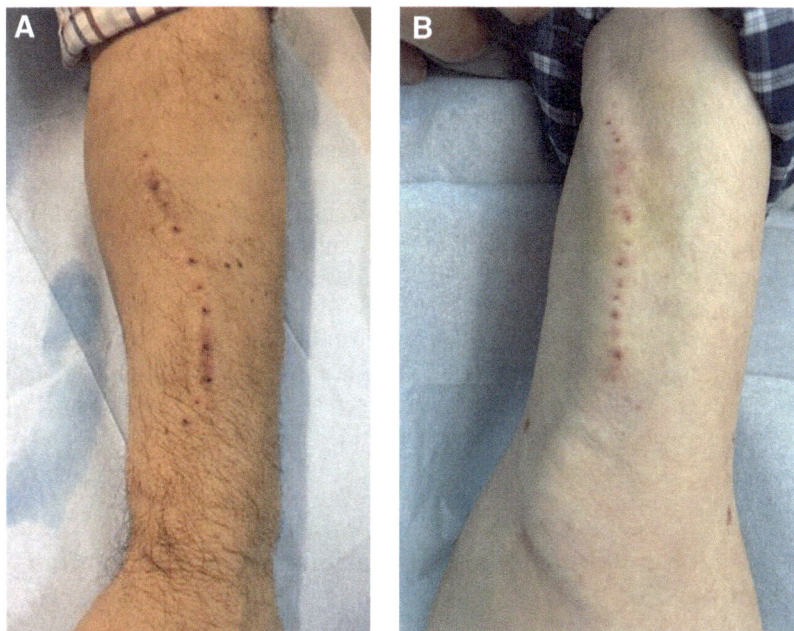

Fig. 1 Rope-ladder technique (A) radiocephalic AVF and (B) brachiobasilic AVF

no digital pressure should be applied until the needle is completely removed (Pinto et al. 2022). The same nephrologist nurse in charge of access cannulation should also remove the needles.

Haemostasis at the cannulation sites should be carried out with gentle pressure in order to prevent blood loss and not to obstruct blood flow completely. The thrill and bruit of the AVF should be continuously perceptible below and above compression (Sousa 2012).

The process of haemostasis can be carried out using dynamic or static pressure (Sousa 2009, 2012; Sousa et al. 2023). Dynamic pressure haemostasis is performed by the patient for 10–15 minutes, with different pressures over time. At the start of the process, the patient performs haemostasis with a higher pressure which decreases over time until it approaches 10–15 minutes. During this process, pressure must be continuous with no interruptions or "visualizations" in order to promote clot formation.

The patient should be trained and instructed on the importance of a correct haemostasis. Once the needle has been removed, the patient should place the thumb on the puncture site and the remaining fingers on the back of the arm/forearm, wrapping it in a "C" shape (Sousa 2009). This way of positioning the fingers limits accidental movement of the dressings from the puncture site, minimizing the risk of bleeding. Bearing in mind that there is a difference between the skin hole and the vessel hole (they don't completely overlap), pressure during haemostasis is exerted on the skin hole in the direction in which the needle was placed. With this technique of dynamic pressure, haemostasis should first be removed from the venous needle and, once haemostasis is complete, the arterial needle should also be removed (Sousa 2009). This strategy makes it possible not to increase the intra-access pressure when removing the arterial needle and thus avoid haemorrhage from the venous site.

Static-pressure haemostasis uses fistula clamps, but they are not recommended as they can cause thrombosis and/or damage the access by excessive pressure during the haemostasis process. Haemostasis of the first cannulation should be carried out by a nephrologist nurse, due to the fragility of the vascular wall and the risk of subcutaneous haematoma formation. Patients should be encouraged to perform one haemostasis at a time, i.e., not both at the same time.

It is important to bear in mind that haemostasis time is different for each AVF. The periodic occurrence of prolonged haemostasis times (longer than 20 minutes) in non-complex cannulations may indicate an increase in intra-access pressure, which could be a sign of dysfunction (Sousa et al. 2023).

2 Decision-making Models for the Selection of Cannulation Techniques

Models allow a critical analysis of clinical data, guiding professionals to make decisions based on scientific evidence and increasing the accuracy and effectiveness of decision-making. Implementation of clinical decision models is key in order to improving care practice. Not only do they promote a systematic, evidence-based approach, but they also reduce errors, improve team communication, and use emerging technologies to optimize patient care. Such factors translate into safer, more effective, and patient-centred care.

Clinical decision-making, particularly when selecting the cannulation technique for an AVF, is fundamental to guaranteeing the success of the procedure and the longevity of the fistula, as well as minimizing complications such as thrombosis, stenosis, and haematomas. The use of clinical decision-making models can help healthcare professionals, especially nephrologist nurses, choose the appropriate puncture technique based on objective criteria that are tailored to the patient (Sousa et al. 2024).

In 2015, the British Society of Nephrology and the Vascular Access Society of Great Britain and Ireland created MAGIC (Managing Access by Generating Improvements in Cannulation), with the aim of exploring and implementing improvements in haemodialysis vascular access care for haemodialysis across the United Kingdom. The "Managing Access by Generating Improvements in Cannulation" model promotes a systematic, evidence-based approach to improving cannulation practice, based on the consensus of experts who are members of the expert group (Fielding et al. 2021). The MAGIC group recommends that any given person should have the opportunity to get involved with self-care of their vascular access as early as possible.

In 2023, Pinto et al. described the nursing consultation concerning the first vascular access cannulation as centred on a decision-making model for AVF cannulation (Pinto et al. 2023). This is an important model regarding physical examination of an AVF, ultrasound, evaluation of needle fear, infection risk, and cannulation technique. Such a structure can help the nurse identify the appropriate cannulation technique according to the AVF's physical and ultrasound characteristics and the patient's concerns (Pinto et al. 2023).

In 2023, Sousa et al. introduced a decision-making model for choosing the appropriate cannulation technique adapted to the patient's characteristics (hygiene self-care profile, patient conditions, and patient decision), the arteriovenous access (type of arteriovenous access and drainage vein), and the experience of the haemodialysis team (experience of the nursing team on the cannulation technique, nurse/patient ratio, and haemodialysis treatment method) (Sousa et al. 2023).

This model has seven premises that can help nephrology nurses choose the correct cannulation technique for the arteriovenous access (Fig. 2). The first premise is to identify the type of arteriovenous access (AVF or polytetrafluoroethylene (PTFE) graft). The roper-ladder cannulation technique can only be used for grafts whereas the buttonhole technique can only be used for AVFs.

The second premise concerns the length of the AVF drainage vein which can influence the choice of the cannulation technique and should be measured by ultrasound. The roper-ladder technique can only be used in AVF draining veins which are longer than 7 cm. When that length is shorter than 7 cm, the nephrology nurse can choose

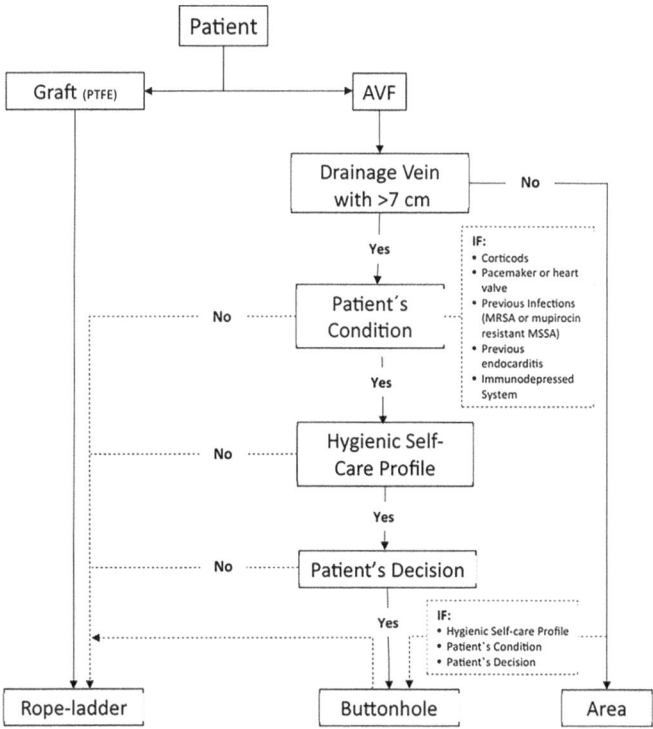

Fig. 2 Cannulation technique decision-making model (Sousa et al. 2023)

between the area or the buttonhole techniques. The choice among these three cannulation techniques depends on the following premises (Sousa et al. 2023).

The third premise is the assessment of the patient's condition, required for the selection of the appropriate cannulation technique. The nephrology nurse should rule out the buttonhole technique in patients with: an increased risk of infection, mainly when corticosteroids or immunosuppressants are being used; a pacemaker or heart valve; a history of previous infections (MRSA) or previous endocarditis; immunosuppressed systems (Sousa et al. 2023). The fourth premise that can influence whether the buttonhole technique is chosen or not is the patient's hygiene care profile. The nephrology nurse must assess such a dimension in order to adapt the technique to this premise. If the patient has problems with his/her hygiene care profile, the nephrology nurse should choose the area or ladder cannulation technique.

The patient's decision concerning the cannulation technique must be considered and, at the same time, he/she must be co-responsible for all aspects associated with such a choice (Sousa et al. 2023). This is the fifth premise.

The sixth and seventh premises concern, respectively, the nursing team's experience of the cannulation technique and the choice of haemodialysis treatment method, which must be considered in order to provide the team with the necessary skills to choose an appropriate cannulation technique.

3 New Approach to Defining Cannulation Techniques

The cannulation technique plays a crucial role in maintaining the patency and functionality of the arteriovenous access and must be adapted to the patient's anatomical characteristics and clinical needs.

Traditionally, three techniques have been considered for AVF cannulation (area cannulation, buttonhole cannulation, and rope-ladder cannulation). However, the evolution of clinical practice and the increasing anatomical complexity of the AVF have highlighted the importance of a complementary approach based on the number of cannulation points used in each HD session. The approach based on the number of cannulation points for each session enables the cannulation technique to be tailor-made and adjusted to the specificities of the access. We propose a two-point classification:

1. Single-site Puncture
   It is characterized by the consistent use of the same arterial and venous puncture sites for each dialysis session (one arterial point and one venous point). The buttonhole cannulation can be performed with either blunt or sharp needles (Staaf et al. 2021).
2. Multi-site Puncture
   It is characterized by the use of at least two distinct puncture points for the arterial and venous needles, with rotation of the sites depending on the vein segment or treatment days. This approach can be broken down as:

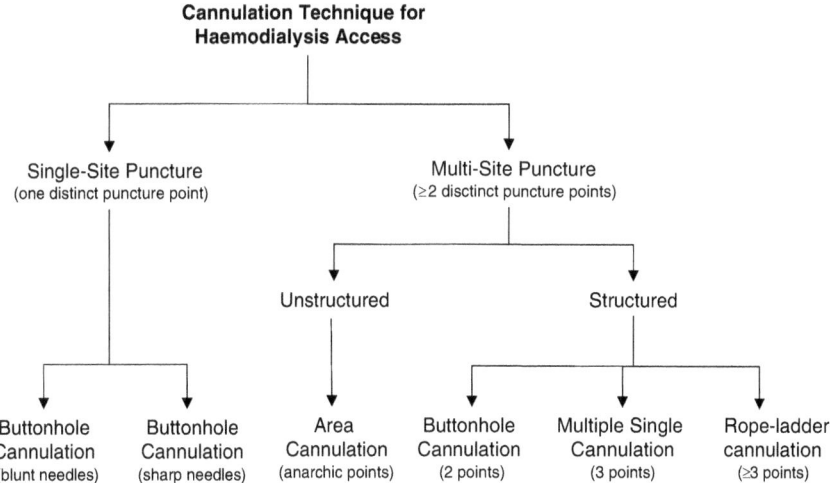

Fig. 3 Definition of cannulation technique

- Unstructured: puncture is performed at multiple points within a limited area without following a fixed pattern or specific sequence, allowing free variation in the choice of puncture sites (Sousa et al. 2023).
- Structured: puncture is performed at predefined and organized points according to a specific pattern, such as rope-ladder (Sousa et al. 2023), buttonhole (Twardowski 2015), or multiple single cannulation (MUST) (Peralta et al. 2021), aiming to preserve the integrity of the fistula and facilitate healing of the puncture sites (Fig. 3).

The choice of the number of puncture sites should be based on prior ultrasound assessment, the anatomical characteristics of the AVF, and patient preference, in order to optimize the longevity of the vascular access and reduce long-term complications.

This new technical definition based on the number of puncture sites does not replace traditional approaches but complements them, providing healthcare professionals with an additional tool to customize the puncture strategy according to the anatomical characteristics of the AVF, patient needs, and clinical recommendations. Its adoption may help optimize AVF preservation and improve the quality of life of patients undergoing haemodialysis.

4 Practical Implications

Decision models are generally based on up-to-date guidelines and clinical evidence, which means that decisions are supported by recognized best practice. It is possible to standardize the choice of the puncture technique based on guidelines and evidence by using decision models, thus enabling nephrology nurses to have a consistent approach based on the best practice. The use of such models to choose the arteriovenous fistula puncture technique provides safer, more effective and personalized care, increasing the longevity of the vascular access, reducing complications, and improving the patient's dialysis experience.

References

Akyol Durmaz A, Mertbilek A, Kara L, Karadeniz D (2015) Determination of the effect of access techniques used during arteriovenous fistula cannulation procedure on pain level. J Nephrol Nurs 10:10–18

Brouwer D (2011) Cannulation camp: basic needle cannulation training for dialysis staff. Dial Transplant 40(10):427–472, E1–E5

Bushey M (2020) Buttonhole cannulation of arteriovenous fistulas: a dialysis nurse's perspective. KIDNEY360 1:279–280

Crespo R (1994) Influence of bevel position of the needle on puncture pain in hemodialysis. J Eur Dial Transpl Nurs Assoc 4:21–23

Crespo Montero R, Rivero Arellano F, Contreras Abad M, Martínez Gomez A, Fuentes Gal M (2004) Pain degree and skin damage during arterio-venous fistula puncture. EDTNA ERCA J 30:208–212

Dinwiddie L, Ball L, Brouwer D, Doss-McQuitty S, Holland J (2013) What nephrologists need to know about vascular access cannulation. Semin Dial 26(3):315–322

Fielding C, Oliver S, Swain A, Gagen A, Kattenhorn S, Waters D et al (2021) Managing access by generating improvements in cannulation: a national quality improvement project. J Vasc Access 22(3):450–456

Gaspar L, Moreira N, Moutinho A, Pinto P, Lima H, Rodrigues F (2003) Puncture of the arterio-venous fistula: bevel upward or bevel downward?. EDTNA ERCA J 29:104

Karkhah S, Pourshaikhian M, Vajargah P, Mahdiabadi M, Mollaei A, Maroufizadeh S et al (2023) Needle direction and distance of arteriovenous fistula cannulation in hemodialysis adequacy; a systematic review and meta-analysis. Arch Acad Emerg Med 11(1):e39

Mehta H, Deabreu D, McDougall J, Goldstein M (2002) Correction of discrepancy between prescribed and actual blood flow rates in chronic hemodialysis patients with use of larger gauge needles. Am J Kidney Dis 39(6):1231–1235

Mondueri A, Calero E, Arce A, Ramón M (2006) Efecto del calibre de la aguja sobre la eficacia de la hemodiálisis. Rev Soc Esp Enferm Nefrol 9(2):128–131

Nesrallah G (2016) Pro: buttonhole cannulation of arteriovenous fistulae. Nephrol Dial Transplant 31:520–523

Ozen N, Tosun B, Sayilan A, Eyileten T, Ozen V, Ecder T et al (2022) Effect of the arterial needle bevel position on puncture pain and postremoval bleeding time in hemodialysis patients: a self-controlled, single-blind study. Hemodial Int 26(4):503–508

Peralta R, Fazendeiro MJ, Carvalho H (2021) Safe needling of arteriovenous fistulae in patients on hemodialysis: literature review and a new approach. Nephrol Nurs J 48(2):169–176

Pinto R, Sousa C, Salgueiro A, Fernandes I (2022) Arteriovenous fistula cannulation in hemodialysis: a vascular access clinical practice guidelines narrative review. J Vasc Access 23(5):825–831

Pinto R, Duarte F, Mata F, Sousa C, Salgueiro A, Fernandes I (2023) Arteriovenous fistula cannulation in hemodialysis: constructing and validating a decision-making model. Revista de Enfermagem Referência 6(2, Suppl. 1):e22021

Pinto R, Ferreira E, Sousa C, Barros J, Correia A, Silva A et al (2023) Skin pigmentation as landmark for arteriovenous fistula cannulation in hemodialysis. J Vasc Access. https://doi.org/10.1177/11297298231193477

Sousa C (2009) Caring for arteriovenous fistula: from theoretical assumptions to practical contexts. Master's dissertation presented to the Abel Salazar Institute of Biomedical Sciences of the University of Porto

Sousa C (2012) Caring for the person arteriovenous fistula: model for continuous improvement. Rev Port Sau Pub 30(1):11–17

Sousa C, Apóstolo J, Figueiredo M, Martins M, Dias V (2013) Physical examination: how to examine the arm with arteriovenous fistula. Hemodial Int 17(2):300–306

Sousa C, Teles P, Ribeiro O, Sousa R, Lira M, Delgado E et al (2023) How to choose the appropriate cannulation technique for vascular access in hemodialysis patients. Ther Apher Dial 27(3):394–401

Sousa C, Teles P, Sousa R, Cabrita F, Ribeiro O, Delgado E et al (2024) Hemodialysis vascular access coordinator: three-level model for access management. Semin Dial 37(2):85–90

Staaf K, Fernström A, Uhlin F (2021) Cannulation technique and complications in arteriovenous fistulas: a Swedish Renal Registry-based cohort study. BMC Nephrol 22:256

Twardowski Z (2015) Update on cannulation techniques. J Vasc Access 16(Suppl 9):S54–S60

van Loon M, Kessel A, van der Sande F, Tordoir J (2009) Cannulation and vascular access-related complications in hemodialysis: factors determining successful cannulation. Hemodial Int 13(4):498–504

Complications in Arteriovenous Fistula Cannulation

Nurten Ozen and Clemente Neves Sousa

Literature shows that nephrology nurses' knowledge, skills, experience, and attitudes toward arteriovenous fistula (AVF) cannulation can influence access complications. Similarly, complications arising from cannulation can have a negative impact on the patient's experience (Wilson et al. 2013; Sousa et al. 2023). A patient with an AVF undergoing dialysis treatment three times a week is subject to 312 cannulations per year (Staaf et al. 2021). Problems are therefore likely to occur during the cannulation process or as a result of needling, including haemorrhage, pain and haematoma, infection, or needling failure. In some patients, such situations can make it difficult to create an AVF due to the fear of complications that may occur and thus delay its creation.

By detecting or identifying situations in which complications associated with cannulation may occur, nephrology nurses can reduce the negative impact on the access as well as on the patient's experience.

1 Haematoma

A haematoma is characterized by the extravasation of blood into the subcutaneous tissue adjacent to the AVF, usually as a result of inappropriate cannulation or transfixation of the posterior wall during cannulation. It can also occur as a result of involuntary

N. Ozen (✉)
Faculty of Nursing, Department of Internal Medicine Nursing, Istanbul University, Istanbul, Turkey
e-mail: nurten.ozen@istanbul.edu.tr

C. N. Sousa
Nursing School of University of Porto, Porto, Portugal
e-mail: clementesousa@esenf.pt

RISE – Health, University of Porto, Porto, Portugal

© The Author(s), under exclusive license to Springer Nature Switzerland AG 2025
N. Ozen et al. (eds.), *Arteriovenous Fistula Management*,
https://doi.org/10.1007/978-3-032-04771-7_7

movement by the patient during hemodialysis (HD), when removing the needle or during the hemostasis process. Such an accumulation of blood outside the vessel can lead to compression of the draining vein, reducing blood flow and increasing the risk of thrombosis. Clinically, this condition is manifested by a painful area that is hard and warm on palpation, with a purplish color around the puncture site and edema.

Haematoma can occur in patients undergoing HD treatment during needling, in the course of the treatment or when the needle is removed (Sousa 2012). It is very important to detect such a situation and to develop strategies that can reduce the impact of the haematoma on the following treatment. The nephrology nurse should first massage the area of the haematoma with an ice cube to promote vasoconstriction of the area and reduce subcutaneous infiltration (Sousa 2012). Ice should be applied only after this procedure, but never directly under the area, as described in Chap. 9.

The technique of needle removal is as important as the cannulation technique itself to protect the vascular access site from damage and ensure proper hemostasis (Pinto et al. 2022). The needle should be withdrawn at an angle close to the angle of insertion. After removing the needle, both the skin and the graft or vessel wall at the needle exit sites should be gently pressed, placing the thumb on the puncture site and the remaining fingers on the back of the arm/forearm, wrapping them in a "C" shape, as described in Chap. 6 (Sousa 2012). Until the needle is completely removed, pressure should not be applied to the puncture site in order to prevent damage to the vascular access (Schimidi et al. 2018). During the first three to five cannulations, hemostasis should be carried out by the nurse. The patient must be educated and trained to carry out hemostasis properly (Sousa et al. 2014, 2021, 2022).

The use of clamps to support hemostasis is generally not recommended. If clamps are to be used, they should only be applied while closely monitoring a matured vascular access with sufficient flow, and they should only be used if flow can still be felt in the AVF while the clamp is in place. Dressings should be applied to the cannulation sites but should not encircle the limb to prevent compression of blood flow in the vascular access. Quality of bruit and thrill should be assessed and documented before the patient leaves the dialysis unit. Difficulties in achieving haemostasis during cannulation or after needle removal may indicate venous outflow stenosis in a patient with normal bleeding times (Pinto et al. 2022). If prolonged haemostasis persists, anticoagulation should be reassessed, dynamic venous pressure measurements should be reviewed, and vascular access flow studies should be carried out in order to determine the cause of stenosis (Schimidi et al. 2018; Lok et al. 2020).

2 Cannulation Difficulty

AVF cannulation can be a challenge for nurses and its difficulty can result from vascular morphology problems (tortuous, deep, or bifurcated) and from the problems with the identification of the appropriate cannulation site. The vascular structure can increase the problems and make cannulation more difficult, as described in Chap. 8.

Good cannulation techniques are crucial for proper AVF care. Cannulation can impact both the outcome of the AVF and the patient's experience, so close attention should be paid to the cannulation process (Sousa et al. 2023).

The main goal of AVF care is to maintain a "good cannulation technique" that preserves its function, prevents AVF complications, and enables a quick and easy use (Staaf et al. 2023). A "good cannulation technique" does not necessarily equal a "successful cannulation," as the term "successful cannulation" refers only to a single attempt at needle insertion. Therefore, it is important to acknowledge that successful cannulation can still occur even if the cannulation technique is not the ideal (Pinto et al. 2022). The process involves more than just the act of inserting needles which is the needling procedure.

Ease of cannulation is a fundamental requirement to minimize AVF complications and ensure its viability (Lok et al. 2020; Coventry et al. 2019). While desirable, this ideal can sometimes be challenging to achieve due to various biological and non-biological factors. Cannulation can be difficult at times, requiring multiple attempts and often leading to iatrogenic complications (Coventry et al. 2019). While this is often true for new fistulas, it can also apply to matured ones (van Loon et al. 2010). Deeper fistulas are harder to cannulate than superficial ones. Moreover, underlying anatomical abnormalities within fistulas can lead to difficulties in cannulating both new and matured fistulas. Even the use of pre-operative vascular mapping techniques such as Doppler may not be enough to prevent this outcome.

Successful AVF cannulation is important to minimize access-related complications and enhance its longevity. Difficult or unsuccessful cannulation can lead to poor dialysis blood flow, high venous pressures, inadequate dialysis, poor quality of life, fistula thrombosis, and extravascular haematomas (Coventry et al. 2019; Pinto et al. 2022). The latter two complications can mean an impending or even permanent access loss and further increasing dependence on temporary bridging catheters. The challenging cannulation of an AVF is an overlooked problem in nephrology practice and is an area filled with uncertainties. Its most common causes are stenosis, immature fistula, extremity edema, anatomical abnormalities, or a combination of these factors. Repeated missed fistula cannulation can lead to serious complications such as haematoma (Harwood et al. 2017), infection (Harwood et al. 2017; Polkinghorne et al. 2013; Al-Jaishi et al. 2017), and aneurysm formation (Harwood et al. 2017; Al-Jaishi et al. 2017). This can result in the need for access revision (Al-Jaishi et al. 2017), central venous catheter placement (Harwood et al. 2017), or access loss (Vachharajani 2014; Schinstock et al. 2011).

When an AVF is hard to cannulate, the vascular access should be analyzed in order to try to understand why. If the majority of nurses cannot cannulate the AVF, the problem is the access and not the nursing team. Then, identifying the cause of the cannulation problems is crucial.

3 Bleeding

Bleeding is characterized by haemorrhage that lasts longer than 15 min after the needle is removed during the hemostasis process or that occurs at home (Sousa 2012).

Cannulation techniques can increase bleeding, especially when the nephrology nurse selects area cannulation as the cannulation technique (Sousa 2012; Sousa et al. 2023). Repeated needle punctures in the same sites cause the needles to damage the vein wall over time and cause it to lose elasticity. As a result, thinning of the vessel wall increases the risk of rupture and hemorrhage. Bleeding is a complication that can occur after puncture during the hemostasis process. In addition, the risk of hemorrhage increases whenever dialysis needles are inserted and removed.

In buttonhole cannulation, the risk of hemorrhage can be high in proximal AVFs with outflow problems (cephalic arch stenosis) and high flow (Sousa et al. 2023). Bleeding can occur during HD due to peri-needle bleeding at the end of the HD session or at home.

Literature shows different approaches to minimizing bleeding, but the main one is a correct analysis of the fistula's characteristics and an appropriate cannulation process, as mentioned in Chap. 6. One strategy to reduce the duration of bleeding after needle removal is to cannulate all superficial AVFs at an angle of 25° (McCann et al. 2008).

The choice of aneurysm cannulation or continuous cannulation must be carefully weighed against the risk of increased skin fragility and subsequent hemorrhage. This is due to the narrowing of the vessel wall after the aneurysm, making it more vulnerable to injury and prone to hemorrhage and rupture.

The cannulation process of the AVF prior to HD is an important part of the HD treatment. Successful needling is required to carry out the treatment using an AV access which requires good needle insertion at each HD session. Incorrect techniques can lead to complications including stenosis and aneurysm development, infections, haematoma, pseudoanuerysm, bleeding, and pain.

4 Infection

AVF infection is a serious complication that can jeopardize the vascular access and the patient's general health. Clinically, AVF infection can be characterized by classic signs of inflammation, such as redness, heat, pain, and edema around the cannulation site. There may also be purulent discharge and hardening of the adjacent tissues.

Vascular access infection is the main type of infection in HD patients and is the second leading cause of death, following only cardiovascular diseases (Li and Chow 2012). The majority of infections are primarily caused by gram-positive cocci (*Staphylococcus aureus* 50%–90%, *Staphylococcus epidermis*, *Streptococcus viridans*, and *Streptococcus faecalis*). Gram-negative organisms account for approximately 33% of infections (Li and Chow 2012), triggering a local and systemic inflammatory response.

HD patients have been shown to be carriers of *Staphylococcus aureus* in the nose and skin more frequently than the general population. Therefore, disinfecting the skin before any needling is extremely important and contributes to the risk of access-related infections. Nephrologist nurses should clean the skin with an approved antimicrobial preparation provided by the facility. Various cleansing solutions with different effectiveness and application times are available for access disinfection Chap. 4. Nurse should wear clean gloves for needling. While circular cleaning is generally preferred over the east–west technique, currently there is no strong evidence to support it (Higgins et al. 2008).

Arteriovenous fistula-associated infection is one of the significant complications related to fistulas. A number of studies have reported an increased risk of infection in patients undergoing needling using the buttonhole technique (MacRae et al. 2012; Labriola et al. 2011). Two systematic reviews have shown that the use of the buttonhole technique is associated with cannulation-related infections (Wong et al. 2014; Grudzinski et al. 2013). Such infections ranged from small skin infections at the access site to bacteremia and sepsis. Inappropriate disinfection protocols, such as inadequate scab removal by nursing staff or self-cannulating patients, have been highlighted as a possible reason for increased infection rates (van Loon et al. 2010). Staff retraining on cleaning techniques and scab removal has resulted in lower infection rates (Labriola et al. 2011). Studies have suggested an increased risk associated with the buttonhole cannulation technique for access-related infections (Labriole et al. 2011; van Loon et al. 2010).

Different cannulation techniques have varying degrees of impact on the incidence of complications. Therefore, the choice of cannulation techniques can lead to an increase or decrease in the risk of complications. Guidelines primarily support rope ladder techniques due to their lower infection risk (Lok et al. 2020; Schmidli et al. 2018).

It is important to properly analyze the signs and symptoms of AVF infection so that such a clinical picture is not mistaken for an intraluminal thrombus. Typically, a thrombus that occupies more than 70% of the lumen can present signs and symptoms (redness, edema, and pain) very similar to those of an infection. In this situation, the pain and edema may improve, but the redness usually never disappears completely, as the cause is not the infectious process, but a thrombotic process, which can lead to thrombosis of the AVF, requiring a prompt observation by the vascular access center or the vascular surgeon.

Using a strict aseptic technique to appropriately prepare access sites can minimize contamination and/or access-related infections, and it should be employed for all needling procedures (Ozen et al. 2017). Needling should be avoided particularly in areas with thin, infection-prone skin, and signs of impending rupture. Treatment should involve avoiding needling in that area.

Empirical treatment in all AVF infections should start with broad-spectrum antibiotics and then be tailored according to culture results (Hemodialysis Adequacy 2006 Work Group 2006).

5 Practical Implications

Nephrologist nurse plays a vital role in preventing complications that might arise from cannulation. Therefore, nurses have important responsibilities in this regard. They should possess knowledge of cannulation techniques, have sufficient theoretical and practical knowledge related to AVF examination, possess advanced communication skills, provide patient-centered care, and continuously improve their cannulation skills through methods like simulation and virtual reality applications. Nurses should be encouraged to use ultrasound during cannulation, and they should have mentors to provide support during challenging cannulation procedures.

Before the needling procedure, it is important to gather a patient's history concerning their arteriovenous access. This history should encompass any changes observed since their previous HD session, as well as any issues encountered during those sessions. Difficulties with inserting needles, clot aspiration, and extended bleeding can all serve as indications of potential complications in the arteriovenous access. It is recommended that nephrology nurses possess an understanding of the indicators of a declining access function and integrate them into their routine vessel assessments. These indicators encompass: alterations in arterial/venous pressures; decreased or disrupted blood flow rate; lowered Kt/V or urea reduction ratio; challenges with needle insertion; and prolonged bleeding.

References

Al-Jaishi A, Liu A, Lok C, Zhang J, Moist L (2017) Complications of the arteriovenous fistula: a systematic review. J Am Soc Nephrol 28:1839–1850

Coventry LL, Hosking JM, Chan DT, Coral E, Lim WH, Towell-Barnard A et al (2019) Variables associated with successful vascular access cannulation in hemodialysis patients: a prospective cohort study. BMC Nephrol 20(1):197. https://doi.org/10.1186/s12882-019-1373-3

Grudzinski A, Mendelssohn D, Pierratos A, Nesrallah G (2013) A systematic review of buttonhole cannulation practices and outcomes. Semin Dial 26(4):465–475. https://doi.org/10.1111/sdi.12116

Harwood L, Wilson B, Goodman M (2017) Cannulation outcomes of the arteriovenous fistula for hemodialysis: a scoping review. Nephrol Nurs J 44:411–426

Hemodialysis Adequacy 2006 Work Group (2006) Clinical practice guidelines for hemodialysis adequacy, update 2006. Am J Kidney Dis 48(Suppl 1):S2–S90. https://doi.org/10.1053/j.ajkd.2006.03.051

Higgins M, Evans DS (2008) Nurses' knowledge and practice of vascular access infection control in haemodialysis patients in the Republic of Ireland. J Ren Care 34(2):48–53. https://doi.org/10.1111/j.1755-6686.2008.00016.x

Labriola L, Crott R, Desmet C, Andre G, Jadoul M (2011) Infectious complications following conversion to buttonhole cannulation of native arteriovenous fistulas: a quality improvement report. Am J Kidney Dis 57:442e8

Li PK, Chow KM (2012) Infectious complications in dialysis—epidemiology and outcomes. Nat Rev Nephrol 8:77–88

Lok CE, Huber TS, Lee T, Shenoy S, Yevzlin AS, Abreo K et al (2020) KDOQI Clinical Practice Guideline for Vascular Access: 2019 update. Am J Kidney Dis 75(4Suppl 2):S1–S164. https://doi.org/10.1053/j.ajkd.2019.12.001

MacRae JM, Ahmed SB, Atkar R, Hemmelgarn BR (2012) A randomized trial comparing buttonhole with rope ladder needling in conventional hemodialysis patients. Clin J Am Soc Nephrol CJASN 7:1632–1638

McCann M, Einarsdóttir H, Van Waeleghem JP, Murphy F, Sedgewick J (2008) Vascular access management 1: an overview. J Ren Care 34(2):77–84. https://doi.org/10.1111/j.1755-6686.2008.00022.x

Ozen N, Tosun N, Cinar FI, Bagcivan G, Yilmaz MI, Askin D et al (2017) Investigation of the knowledge and attitudes of patients who are undergoing hemodialysis treatment regarding their arteriovenous fistula. J Vasc Access 18(1):64–68. https://doi.org/10.5301/jva.5000618

Pinto R, Sousa C, Salgueiro A, Fernandes I (2022) Arteriovenous fistula cannulation in hemodialysis: a vascular access clinical practice guidelines narrative review. J Vasc Access 23(5):825–831

Polkinghorne KR, Chin GK, MacGinley RJ, Owen AR, Russell C, Talaulikar GS et al (2013) KHA-CARI guideline: vascular access – central venous catheters, arteriovenous fistulae and arteriovenous grafts. Nephrology 18:701–705

Schinstock C, Albright R, Williams A, Dillon J, Berfstralh E, Jenson B et al (2011) Outcomes of arteriovenous fistula creation after the Fistual first initiative. Clin J Am Soc Nephrol 6:1996–2002

Schmidli J, Widmer MK, Basile C, de Donato G, Gallieni M, Gibbons CP et al (2018) Editor's Choice - Vascular Access: 2018 Clinical Practice Guidelines of the European Society for Vascular Surgery (ESVS). Eur J Vasc Endovasc Surg 55(6):757–818. https://doi.org/10.1016/j.ejvs.2018.02.001

Sousa C (2012) Caring for the person arteriovenous fistula: model for continuous improvement. Rev Port Sau Pub 30(1):11–17

Sousa C, Apóstolo J, Figueiredo M, Martins M, Dias V (2013) Physical examination: how to examine the arm with arteriovenous fistula. Hemodial Int 17(2):300–306

Sousa C, Apóstolo J, Figueiredo M, Martins M, Dias V (2014) Interventions to promote self-care of people with arteriovenous fistula. J Clin Nurs 23(13-14):1796–1802

Sousa C, Paquete A, Teles P, Pinto C, Dias V, Ribeiro O et al (2021) Investigating the effect of a structured intervention on the development of self-care behaviors with arteriovenous fistula in hemodialysis patients. Clin Nurs Res 30(6):866–874

Sousa C, Teles P, Paquete A, Dias V, Manzini C, Nicole A et al (2022) Effects of demographic and clinical character on differences in self-care behavior levels with arteriovenous fistula by hemodialysis patients: an ordinal logistic regression approach. Ther Apher Dial 26(5):992–998

Sousa C, Teles P, Ribeiro O, Sousa R, Lira M, Delgado E et al (2023) How to choose the appropriate cannulation technique for vascular access in hemodialysis patients. Ther Apher Dial 27(3):394–401

Staaf K, Fernström A, Uhlin F (2021) Cannulation technique and complications in arteriovenous fistulas: a Swedish Renal Registry-based cohort study. BMC Nephrol 22(1):256. https://doi.org/10.1186/s12882-021-02458-z

Staaf K, Fernström A, Uhlin F (2023) Preconditions that facilitate cannulation in arteriovenous fistula: a mixed-methods study. J Ren Care 49(4):264–277. https://doi.org/10.1111/jorc.12448

Vachharajani T (2014) The role of cannulation and fistula care. Semin Dial 28:24–27

van Loon MM, Goovaerts T, Kessels AG, van der Sande FM, Tordoir JH (2010) Buttonhole needling of haemodialysis arteriovenous fistulae results in less complications and interventions compared to the rope-ladder technique. Nephrol Dial Transplant 25:225e30

Wilson B, Harwood L, Oudshoorn A (2013) Moving beyond the "perpetual novice": understanding the experiences of novice hemodialysis nurses and cannulation of the arteriovenous fistula. CANNT J 23(1):11–18

Wong B, Muneer M, Wiebe N, Storie D, Shurraw S, Pannu N et al (2014) Buttonhole versus rope-ladder cannulation of arteriovenous fistulas for hemodialysis: a systematic review. Am J Kidney Dis 64(6):918–936. https://doi.org/10.1053/j.ajkd.2014.06.018

Xi W, Harwood L, Diamant MJ, Brown JB, Gallo K, Sontrop JM et al (2011) Patient attitudes towards the arteriovenous fistula: a qualitative study on vascular access decision making. Nephrol Dial Transplant 26(10):3302–3308. https://doi.org/10.1093/ndt/gfr055

Ultrasound for the Arteriovenous Fistula

Clemente Neves Sousa, Nurten Ozen, Paulo Teles, Tanju Kisbet, and Volkan Ozen

The application of ultrasound in the arteriovenous access has acquired increasing relevance in the context of haemodialysis, in particular for the dialysis team (nephrology nurses and nephrologists). Its relevance is directly related to the ability to provide fast and accurate information in real time, enabling agile and well-founded decisions to be made. Furthermore, its importance is related to the ability to provide detailed information on the vascular anatomy (arterial and venous), on changes in vessel morphology or on the structure and access flow, contributing to early detection of complications and optimization of patient care (Zamboli et al. 2014; Norton de Matos et al. 2023).

C. N. Sousa (✉)
Nursing School of University of Porto, Porto, Portugal
e-mail: clementesousa@esenf.pt

RISE – Health, University of Porto, Porto, Portugal

N. Ozen
Faculty of Nursing, Department of Internal Medicine Nursing, Istanbul University, Istanbul, Turkey
e-mail: nurten.ozen@istanbul.edu.tr

P. Teles
School of Economics, University of Porto, Porto, Portugal
e-mail: pteles@fep.up.pt

LIAAD-INESC Porto LA, Porto, Portugal

T. Kisbet
Prof. Dr. Cemil Tascioglu City Hospital, Department of Radiology, Istanbul, Turkey
e-mail: tanjukisbet@hotmail.com

V. Ozen
Prof. Dr. Cemil Tascioglu City Hospital, Department of Anesthesiology and Reanimation, Istanbul, Turkey
e-mail: vozen81@gmail.com

© The Author(s), under exclusive license to Springer Nature Switzerland AG 2025
N. Ozen et al. (eds.), *Arteriovenous Fistula Management*,
https://doi.org/10.1007/978-3-032-04771-7_8

Ultrasound is an indispensable tool for nephrology nurses to provide greater safety, precision, and efficiency in vascular access care, preventing complications and ensuring the patient receives the highest-quality haemodialysis treatment. Ultrasound can be used by nephrology nurses in the dialysis team to assess the morphology and vascular structure of the vessels in the arteriovenous fistula (AVF) as an aid to safe cannulation, continuous monitoring, and surveillance of the AVF, but that requires training.

Nephrology nurses should include ultrasound in their daily practice in order to play a more proactive and relevant role in promoting the health and well-being of patients with end-stage renal diseases.

1 Morphology and Vascular Structure of the Arteriovenous Fistula

Assessment of the morphology and vascular structure of the AVF by ultrasound is essential to ensure the success of the cannulation procedure and the patency of the fistula. This assessment makes it possible to observe the morphology of the vessel, detect changes in the vessel's structures, and analyse the flow and identify complications, and is essential for monitoring the maturation process and surveillance of the fistula (Table 1).

The vascular morphology of the fistula is related to the external characteristics and general shape of the drainage vein, considering: the shape, that is, the configuration of the drainage vein (straight, tortuous, dilated, or narrow); the size (diameter of the vein); and continuity of the drainage vein (length, bifurcation, presence of irregularities, or identification of thrombus). Morphology concerns the "shape" and "general appearance" of veins when scanned by ultrasound. By analysing the morphology, it is possible to understand the general configuration of the fistula, such as diameter and type of anastomosis, dilation of the drainage vein, and absence of visible obstructions.

Assessment of the vascular morphology enables measuring the anastomosis size, which should be between 3 mm and 4 mm, and the identification of the anastomosis type, whether it is side-to-side or side-to-end (Norton de Matos et al. 2023). Detecting

Table 1 Issues concerning the arteriovenous fistula to be scanned by ultrasound

Vascular morphology (vessel external characteristics)	**Vascular structure** (vessel internal characteristics)
Configuration of the drainage vein (straight, tortuous, dilated, or narrow)	Wall thickness (thickening of the media layer of the vessel)
Size (diameter of the vein)	Wall texture (detection of calcifications, fibrosis, or intrinsic lesions)
Continuity of the drainage vein (length, bifurcation, presence of irregularities, or identification of thrombus)	Vessel layers (adventitia, media and intima)
	Presence of abnormalities (endothelial problems, intraluminal material, or changes in wall elasticity)

the reduction or narrowing of the juxta-anastomotic vein, as well as a tortuous segment, is very important. The drainage vein must be visible, with a diameter between 5 mm and 6 mm, straight, without tortuosity or dilations (Ibeas et al. 2017). The presence of irregularities and vascular-structure problems must be carefully detected because they can influence the maturation process and delay or prevent using the fistula for haemodialysis treatment. Ultrasound is the appropriate method for assessing intraluminal thrombi, allowing a detailed analysis of their morphological characteristic impact (Teodorescu et al. 2012; Voiculescu and Hentschel 2021). Intraluminal thrombi can present different echogenic, varyng according to their stage of evolution. Recent thrombi are hypoechoic (poorly reflective), while organized or older thrombi are hyperechoic (hyperreflective) due to fibrotic organization (Zamboli et al. 2014). It is important to identify the anatomical location (arterial or venous cannulation, drainage vein, or other location), the degree of occlusion (partial or total), the adherence of the thrombus to the vascular wall (very adherent thrombi suggest chronicity), and the longitudinal lenght of the thrombus. This information can be provided by ultrasound through B mode. However, during the evaluation of intraluminal thrombi, it is important to study the impact of thrombi on the fistula blood flow. Flow absence in a region occupied by thrombi suggests complete obstruction. The presence of residual flow around the thrombus, either above or below it, accompained by turbulence, suggests a partial occlusion associated with stenosis. Assessment of blood flow in the brachial artery can provide relevant information about the impact of thrombi on the fistula. Detailed ultrasound assessment of intraluminal thrombus is crucial to determine the severity of the intervention and guide clinical interventions, ensuring fistula patency. The information provided by the assessment of the vascular morphology through ultrasound can help the nephrology nurse plan the cannulation sites and needle direction (anterograde or retrograde) (Sousa et al. 2023).

The fistula's vascular structure is related to the internal characteristics and composition of the vessel walls, considering: wall thickness, that is, observation of changes in the level of thickening of the media layer of the vessel; wall texture (detection of calcifications, fibrosis, or intrinsic lesions); vessel layers, that is, visualization of the integrity of the different layers (adventitia, media, and intima); and presence of abnormalities (identification of thrombus, endothelial problems, intraluminal material, or changes in wall elasticity). The structure is more related to the internal "composition" and "integrity" of the vessel. Thus, it allows determining the quality of the vessel, checking for the presence of thickening, thrombi, calcifications, or any condition that could compromise the function of the vessel, which hinders puncturing or the blood flow.

Assessment of the fistula's vascular structure is important for the success of haemodialysis treatment and access patency. Changes in the vascular structure can compromise flow and lead to dysfunction and thrombosis. The feeding artery usually has a lumen with well-defined and uniform walls, without irregularities or thickenings and calcifications. The diameter can vary between 2 mm and 4 mm, depending on the selected artery (radial or brachial respectively). Flow is assessed in the brachial artery whose flow resistance is low, with a systolic peak between 100 cm/s and 400 cm/s and resistance index <0.7 (Norton de Matos et al. 2023). Usually, the flow in the anastomosis is accelerated and turbulent due to the passage of blood from the high-pressure (arterial) system to the low-pressure (venous) system.

The passage of flow from the artery to the vein causes the vein diameter to increase between 5 mm and 6 mm and leads to changes in the vein wall, mainly the thickening of the media layer of the vein. The wall of the drainage vein must not show any signs of excessive thickening, narrowing, or irregularities that could compromise the fistula's regular functioning. The flow in the drainage vein is continuous and has high speed, with no interruptions or significant turbulence in the anterograde direction.

In the course of the drainage-route assessment using ultrasound, the identification of changes in the texture of the vein wall is key, that is, detection of sites with inappropriate focal diameter or venous segments with fibrosis. Such changes can provide crucial information about the fistula's maturation and possible success.

Inspecting the integrity of the vessel layers with ultrasound is very helpful in the detection of an aneurysm or pseudoaneurysm in the fistula. Aneurysms are focal and permanent dilations of the vessel resulting from the weakening of the vascular wall. Typically, such dilations occur due to factors associated with chronic increase of the flow, systematic cannulation in the same area or changes in the elasticity of the vascular wall. When the structure of the vein is analysed by ultrasound, the wall remains intact (all three layers are present) with well-defined contours showing only the vein dilation. The flow is normally turbulent and slow inside the aneurysm and continuous and normal outside it.

Pseudoaneurysms are characterized by the rupture of the vessel wall, resulting in the formation of a cavity filled with blood, delimited by adjacent tissues and not by all the layers of the vascular wall (Teodorescu et al. 2012). This condition is generally associated with systematic cannulation at the same site and vascular trauma. Pseudoaneurysms have different ultrasound characteristics from aneurysms. A pseudoaneurysm usually presents an oval structure adjacent to the main vessel, with irregular contours and not circumscribed by a true vascular wall (Voiculescu and Hentschel 2021). When the flow is assessed, it shows the "ying-yang" sign, which reflects the bidirectional flow typical of pseudoaneurysms.

Differentiating between aneurysms and pseudoaneurysms is essential for carrying out appropriate therapeutic planning tailored to each condition. Aneurysms can be monitored clinically while pseudoaneurysms generally require intervention due to the increased risk of rupture, thrombosis, or compression of adjacent structures (Norton de Matos et al. 2023). The use of ultrasound is essential to assess the colour flow and vascular structure of the vessel, enabling an accurate diagnosis and the implementation of appropriate strategies.

The use of ultrasound in daily practice makes it possible to identify situations that would otherwise be underestimated or inadequately diagnosed. The presence of these anomalous situations cannot promote fistula patency, particularly synechiae.

Endothelial problems can compromise permeability of the fistula. The existence of synechiae can cause a focal decrease in vessel diameter, leading to stenosis (Norton de Matos et al. 2023; Chaudhary et al. 2025). It is important to map the entire path of the fistula, from the arterial segment, anastomosis, juxta-anastomosis, and drainage vein in order to identify locations with reduced diameter and compatible with stenosis.

The use of ultrasound enables assessment of the decrease in the luminal diameter, identification of the thickening of the vessel wall, and evaluation of the pattern and characteristics of flow at the site of stenosis (increase in systolic peak, turbulence or flow disturbances, and pre-stenosis, stenosis and post-stenosis). Stenosis can occur in different parts of the fistula and therefore can be rated as inflow, midflow, or outflow stenosis, Chap. 4. The information provided by ultrasound must be correlated with the clinical signs of the physical examination, with the functional parameters of the fistula and with the parameters that result from the interaction between the fistula and the monitor.

2 Safe Cannulation of the Arteriovenous Fistula

Cannulation of arteriovenous fistulas is a complex and challenging process that requires high technical precision and in-depth knowledge of the anatomy and physiology of the vascular access (Pinto et al. 2022). Nephrology nurses must understand the importance and master the use of ultrasound in clinical practice, as it allows for a faster, more accurate, and accessible approach to detecting problems/complications and planning care. The application of this technology should not just be for needling, but should be considered a very important tool to improve decision-making regarding fistula cannulation (Sousa et al. 2023).

The use of ultrasound allows real-time scanning of the vascular network and haemodynamic characteristics, enabling a detailed assessment of the draining vein (Iglesias et al. 2021). Ultrasound has proved to be an important tool in assessing and scanning the vascular morphology, allowing a more detailed assessment of the characteristics of the fistula such as, in particular: diameter of the vein; sites with reduced diameter; depth; bifurcations of the draining vein; location of the anastomosis; and degree of maturation. This analysis makes it possible to optimize the fistula needling process.

Identification of morphological changes in the drainage vein that may compromise or make cannulation difficult is very important. The length of such vein must be determined and the presence of bifurcation must be detected, as well as the diameter along the entire length of the vein. Ultrasound can help finding tortuous segments of the vein that may not be visible and should be avoided as needling sites or as areas of bifurcation. Ultrasound allows to determine the exact depth of the vein, to adjust the needle angle for cannulation and the cannulation technique (Sousa et al. 2013, 2023). It is then possible to identify the ideal location or segment for needling, reducing the risk of complications such as infiltrations or haematomas. Such information allows individualized planning according to the individual characteristics of the patient and of the access drainage vein, promoting safe practice, reducing the risk of complications, avoiding damage to the vessel structure, and optimizing results (Pinto et al. 2023; Sousa et al. 2023).

Ultrasound is a very important tool to assess the structure of the vein, particularly the thickness of the wall. With the creation of the fistula, the draining vein undergoes adaptive changes, namely hypertrophy of the middle layer (Chaudhary et al. 2025). Under normal conditions, the vein has a wall with homogeneous echogenicity, without interruptions or areas of hypo or hyperechogenicity. This analysis of the vein makes it possible to identify where the wall is thicker to withstand needling or where it is more fragile, in order to avoid needling.

Detection of changes in the wall is often associated with pathological problems such as intimal hyperplasia, enabling the identification of areas with reduced diameter (Iglesias et al. 2021). This analysis, made with ultrasound, allows these areas to be avoided and enhances the success of cannulation. Ultrasound can help detecting the presence of synechiae and avoid needling in these areas.

Ultrasound enables to check whether it is an aneurysm or a pseudoaneurysm and to select the appropriate locations, avoiding the pseudoaneurysm. In the presence of a pseudoaneurysm, referral to a vascular access centre or vascular surgeon is required. Another important aspect to be detected by ultrasound is the presence of thrombi which enables the nephrology nurse to seek another site for needle insertion or to scan the patent lumen (without thrombus) in order to select the needle site and direction. Ultrasound helps in defining the best location for needle insertion and avoid cannulation failures.

Cannulation of the fistula can be challenging for the nephrology nurse, especially when the vein is deep, difficult to palpate or tortuous, in patients with anatomical changes, obesity, oedema, or complications such as thrombi or stenosis. Ultrasound-guided or -assisted cannulation may bring benefits in terms of safety, efficiency, and fistula preservation for these specific situations (Iglesias et al. 2021).

The ultrasound-guided cannulation is characterized by the use of ultrasound throughout the needling procedure. In this method, the nurse uses the probe to identify the precise location of the vein and to visualise the needle in real time as it advances, allowing high accuracy during insertion. This real-time scanning minimizes the risk of complications such as haematomas or unintended perforation. Ultrasound-guided cannulation is particularly valuable in difficult vascular accesses and newly created fistulas, where increased precision is essential. In contrast, ultrasound-assisted cannulation involves the use of ultrasound before the needling. The ultrasound is used to assess and select the optimal cannulation site, but the needle is not visualised during insertion, resulting in moderate accuracy compared with the guided approach. This technique is suitable for routine situations and for the preliminary screening of the cannulation site, especially when access conditions are favourable and do not require continuous real-time imaging to achieve successful cannulation.

Ultrasound capability provides detailed information on the vascular morphology and structure which is key for optimizing cannulation, ensuring safe cannulation, and defining the best needling site. Despite the challenges, the benefits are evident and justify the use of this technology in the clinical context as a complement in decision-making for cannulation.

3   Surveillance of the Arteriovenous Fistula

Ultrasonography is a fundamental tool for an accurate and non-invasive assessment of the morphology and structure of the vascular network, as well as the haemodynamic conditions of the fistula.

Maintaining the AVF function depends on careful surveillance and early intervention in cases of dysfunction. Systematic use of ultrasound for surveillance makes it possible to detect alterations that are not yet clinically evident, enabling more assertive decision-making if early intervention or continuous monitoring is required.

Ultrasound surveillance of a fistula means the set of systematic and periodic procedures designed to identify morphological and structural changes at the vascular level in the access. Ultrasound is important for early detecting problems or alterations that can jeopardize the access. This device is very useful during the fistula maturation process to detect stenosis, monitor aneurysms or pseudoaneurysms, identify thrombi, and analyse the flow (Norton de Matos et al. 2023).

Monitoring the maturation process using ultrasound is essential to find out whether the draining vein has the right diameter and flow (Sousa et al. 2013). Ultrasound can assist identifying factors that delay or prevent that maturation such as stenosis, insufficient flow, or anatomical problems that need correction. It is also very important for planning and making clinical decisions during the maturation process in order to begin cannulation.

The main cause of AVF failure is stenosis, usually located in the inflow, midflow, or outflow. This condition can lead to a progressive flow reduction and, consequently, thrombosis of the access. Ultrasound allows the detection of stenoses along the draining artery and vein through the analysis of intraluminal diameter, flow velocity profile at the stenotic site, associated turbulence, and by assessing the efficiency of the AVF and its suitability for haemodialysis. These findings must be correlated with clinical and laboratory data to ensure an accurate diagnosis and an appropriate treatment plan (Norton de Matos et al. 2023).

Ultrasound is very important in the detection of the presence of aneurysms or pseudoaneurysms, as well as their progression. It can accurately measure the diameter of the aneurysm and early detect changes in the structure of the vein, i.e., the integrity of its wall, as well as changes in the vein that indicate an increased risk of complications. This device enables monitoring and surveillance of aneurysms and the detection of pseudo-aneurysms, allowing their referral for intervention before serious complications occur such as rupture or compression of adjacent structures.

Ultrasound evaluation plays an important role in detecting intraluminal thrombi and thrombosis. The echographic identification of intraluminal thrombi allows the determination of the extent and degree of obstruction of the lumen, thus enabling clinical management or the planning of endovascular and/or surgical intervention (Norton de Matos et al. 2023). This approach can improve AVF patency.

The use of ultrasound in haemodialysis units is essential for the management of the arteriovenous access because vascular access monitoring and surveillance programmes are very important. The three-level model (3Level_M) is a vascular management model based on three levels, each one with different training courses aimed at increasing competences and with specific training in a practical context aimed at developing instrumental competences (Sousa et al. 2024). The 3Level_M has different levels of decision-making at each level, defining the flow of information and patient referral. The model includes ultrasound at the three levels with the aim of providing new and/or additional information that can help improve decision-making, Chap. 5. The existence of a vascular-access management programme makes it possible to increase fistula patency, detect complications early, reduce invasive procedures, define the time of intervention, and adjust/customize strategies according to each patient's conditions. The 3LeveL_M includes education and training at each level, with the aim of promoting the development of health professionals in terms of technical skills and decision-making (Sousa et al. 2024).

4 Empowerment of the Nurse

Training nurses with this technology is very important, enabling them to acquire the technical skills, autonomy, and confidence needed to applying ultrasound effectively and safely, which requires a structured training programme and continuing education. The former should include theoretical and practical training, as well as simulation in a clinical context with a workload adjusted to consolidate the required skills.

This process begins with appropriate education and training. Initial training should include theoretical foundations such as the anatomy and physiology of the vascular network, the AVF physiology, the physical principles of ultrasound, and image interpretation (Sousa 2012). Nurses should understand the concepts of frequency, wavelength, depth, and the interaction of ultrasound with biological tissues associated with it. Additionally, knowledge of the different ultrasound modes is required, such as B-mode, colour Doppler, and pulsed wave Doppler, which are key for the assessment of an AVF.

In practice, training should include the acquisition of technical skills in order to manipulate the transducer (transverse and longitudinal mode), select the appropriate parameters on the ultrasound machine, identify vascular structures in B-mode or in colour-Doppler mode, and assess the flow using a pulsed wave Doppler. These skills include measuring the diameter and depth of arterial and venous vessels, detecting problems in the vascular structure, and monitoring the access flow spectrum. It is therefore essential that nurses develop interpretation skills in order to distinguish normal images from pathological findings. It is essential to carry out clinical supervision activities, where nurses can be guided by experts' professionals during the ultrasound examination.

Resource availability, such as high-quality ultrasound equipment and time allocated for training, is fundamental for nurses to be able to include this practice into their work routine. The design of institutional protocols setting the use of ultrasound for the assessment and management of AVFs is also key to provide standardized care and ensure patient safety.

There are, of course, significant challenges in the process of training nurses to use ultrasound in dialysis units, but the potential benefits for patients, professionals, and the dialysis unit as a whole are undeniable. By training nurses in the use of ultrasound, not only do healthcare institutions strengthen their workforce, but also promote a more integrated and efficient approach to the care of haemodialysis patients. Therefore, nurse training should be seen not only as an opportunity, but as an urgent need for the progress of nursing practice and the improvement of health outcomes.

5 Practical Implications

The use of ultrasound in the assessment and treatment of the AVF is an essential tool for improving the quality of nursing care in nephrology. This device enables a detailed analysis of the vascular morphology and structure of the fistula, as well as its application in real time during needling, providing greater safety and reducing the risk of haematoma or infiltration. It is also key for AVF surveillance, enabling early detection of problems and identifying the time for intervention.

Training nurses to use ultrasound is critical in order to maximize the benefits of this technology. Education and training are important to develop skills in ultrasound manipulation, image interpretation, and decision making.

References

Chaudhary SK, Dikshit NA, Yadu N, Parihar A, Kohli N, Dwivedi DK (2025) Efficacy of ultrasonography and color-Doppler for early prediction of hemodialysis arteriovenous fistula unassisted maturation. J Vasc Access 26(5):1495–1503

Ibeas J, Roca-Tey R, Vallespín J, Moreno T, Moñux G, Martí-Monrós A et al (2017) Spanish clinical guidelines on vascular access for haemodialysis. Nefrologia 37(Suppl 1):1–191

Iglesias R, Lodi M, Rubiella C, Parisotto M, Ibeas J (2021) Ultrasound guided cannulation of dialysis access. J Vasc Access 22(1_Suppl):106–112

Norton de Matos A, Sousa C, Teixiera G (2023) Doppler ultrasound in vascular access for haemodialysis. Gráfica de Paredes, Lda, Porto

Pinto R, Sousa C, Salgueiro A, Fernandes I (2022) Arteriovenous fistula cannulation in hemodialysis: a vascular access clinical practice guidelines narrative review. J Vasc Access 23(5):825–831

Pinto R, Ferreira E, Sousa C, Barros J, Correia A, Silva A et al (2023) Skin pigmentation as landmark for arteriovenous fistula cannulation in hemodialysis. J Vasc Access 25(6):1925–1931. https://doi.org/10.1177/11297298231193477

Sousa C (2012) Caring for the person arteriovenous fistula: model for continuous improvement. Rev Port Sau Pub 30(1):11–17

Sousa C, Apóstolo J, Figueiredo M, Martins M, Dias V (2013) Physical examination: how to examine the arm with arteriovenous fistula. Hemodial Int 17(2):300–306

Sousa C, Teles P, Ribeiro O, Sousa R, Lira M, Delgado E et al (2023) How to choose the appropriate cannulation technique for vascular access in hemodialysis patients. Ther Apher Dial 27(3):394–401

Sousa C, Teles P, Sousa R, Cabrita F, Ribeiro O, Delgado E et al (2024) Hemodialysis vascular access coordinator: three-level model for access management. Semin Dial 37(2):85–90

Teodorescu V, Gustavson S, Schanzer H (2012) Duplex ultrasound evaluation of hemodialysis access: a detailed protocol. Int J Nephrol 2012:508956. https://doi.org/10.1155/2012/508956

Voiculescu A, Hentschel D (2021) Point-of-care vascular ultrasound: of fistulas and flows. Adv Chronic Kidney Dis 28(3):227–235

Zamboli P, Fiorini F, D'Amelio A, Fatuzzo P, Granata A (2014) Color Doppler ultrasound and arteriovenous fistulas for hemodialysis. J Ultrasound 17(4):253–263

Self-care Behaviours with the Arteriovenous Fistula

Clemente Neves Sousa, Nurten Ozen, and Paulo Teles

Patients with end-stage renal disease (ESRD) undergoing haemodialysis (HD) need a properly functioning arteriovenous fistula (AVF). Furthermore, they must look after their AVF correctly and take specific care with this type of vascular access. Developing patients' self-care behaviours with such access enables them to maintain the access in the best conditions, reducing thrombosis, and infection.

Scientific literature has shown that the development of self-care behaviours by patients in order to prevent complications or to manage signs and symptoms associated with the vascular access is very important for promoting their quality of treatment and quality of life. However, several studies have also shown that a significant number of patients have low or very low level of self-care behaviours with AVF (Pessoa and Linhares 2015; Sousa et al. 2017; Sousa et al. 2021; Bulbul et al. 2023; Dilbilir and Kavurmaci 2024). Therefore, implementing strategies designed to develop self-care behaviours is very important, but knowing the characteristics of patients with very low self-care level in order to adjust the strategy followed is also required.

C. N. Sousa (✉)
Nursing School of University of Porto, Porto, Portugal
e-mail: clementesousa@esenf.pt

RISE – Health, University of Porto, Porto, Portugal

N. Ozen
Faculty of Nursing, Department of Internal Medicine Nursing, Istanbul University, Istanbul, Turkey
e-mail: nurten.ozen@istanbul.edu.tr

P. Teles
School of Economics, University of Porto, Porto, Portugal
e-mail: pteles@fep.up.pt

LIAAD-INESC Porto LA, Porto, Portugal

1 Self-Care Behaviours With the Arteriovenous Fistula

The patency of an AVF does not depend solely on good surgical construction or on the care taken by the nephrology nurse during HD treatment, but also on the care taken by the patient with such access. Self-care plays a crucial role in this setting and empowering patient to take responsibility for their daily care is a key strategy to extend the lifespan of an AVF and prevent complications.

Sousa (2012) came up with a nursing-care framework that emphasizes patient empowerment and surveillance associated with the process performed by the nurse, Chap. 1. His patient empowerment part is based on Dorothea Orem's Self-Care Theory. Self-care with an AVF must be considered as the set of behaviours intentionally performed by a person in order to maintain health and well-being and promote the patency of the AVF (Sousa et al. 2015a). Any patient carrying out self-care behaviours becomes a self-care agent which leads him/her to develop a set of cognitive, perceptive, and memory capabilities, as well as a set of skills and values that enable him/her to realize the need for self-care (Sousa 2012). Thus, the patient can acquire a set of skills and knowledge that he/she was unaware of and that enable him/her to improve his/her self-care behaviours such as, among others, knowledge related to preserving the vascular network, preventing trauma to the arms, handling needle removal, and maintaining haemostasis or skills required to feel the thrill.

Self-care deficits arise when a person with ESRD is unable to meet the care needs related to the AVF. This may also occur due to incapacity, limitation, lack or mismatch of knowledge, or difficulty in considering the needs of self-care requirements. In other words, there is an imbalance between one's needs to meet his/her self-care requirements and the ability to perform self-care.

Nursing intervention is required at this point in order to help, monitor, make up for, and replace such deficits (Pessoa et al. 2020). The process of self-care behaviours acquisition by these patients is complex and it takes time for the nephrology nurse to identify the difficulties or aspects that may limit such an acquisition. By promoting self-care behaviours with the AVF, the nurse can motivate the patient to acquire the knowledge, capacity, and competence required to improve care with their access (Sousa et al. 2014).

Sousa (2012) identified four temporal dimensions according to the assessment of end-stage renal disease: anticipatory self-care in the creation of the AVF; self-care within 48 h after the creation of the AVF; self-care during the maturation of the AVF; and self-care with the AVF in haemodialysis (Sousa 2012). Each dimension encompasses some knowledge and the acquisition of capabilities and skills that have to be carried out by the patient with the aim of promoting AVF patency and reducing complications.

Anticipatory Self-Care in the Creation of the Arteriovenous Fistula

Patients with terminal ESRD should begin by preserving the vascular network before the creation of the AVF. This dimension corresponds to the time span from chronic kidney disease to AVF creation.

Literature shows that repeated catheterizations are associated with venous network thrombosis, affecting 57% of the cephalic vein, 14% of the basilic vein, and 10% of the brachial vein (Allen et al. 2000). Procedures that may result in thrombosis of the vascular network should be prevented (Sousa et al. 2018; Pessoa et al. 2020). Patients should be encouraged to preserve their vascular network in order to provide appropriate arterial and venous conditions for the creation of the AVF.

In a European study, 85 renal patients, 687 nephrologists, 194 nurses, and 140 surgeons/radiologists compared and analysed their perception regarding the decisions related to the vascular access that deserved priority (van der Veer et al. 2015). Vein preservation was given lower priority by patients than by clinicians and surgeons/radiologists who ranked it in the third and second places, respectively. Nurses ranked vein preservation in the 18th place out of 42 topics related to vascular access (van der Veer et al. 2015). This situation may mean that patients do not usually follow the recommendations and strategy provided by the doctor/nurse for vein preservation.

A study carried out in Portugal with 145 ESRD patients showed that 36.8% of patients carried out self-care behaviours to preserve their vascular network (Sousa et al. 2018). In this study, 109 patients were followed by a nephrologist and 36 were not, and the 2 groups were compared. Patients in the former group (followed by the nephrologist) carried out self-care behaviours more often than those in the latter (59.2 versus 29.4%, respectively, $p < 0.001$). The authors suggest that patients do not understand the importance of preserving their vascular network and its contribution to preventing situations that could compromise the arm veins. They also claim that patients do not "understand" or "value" the recommendations made by nephrologists on the preservation of the vascular network (Hakim and Himmelfarb 2009). This finding means that the patients involved in these studies did not follow or had difficulty following the recommended guidelines.

The results reported in these articles show that a large number of patients do not value or do not perform self-care behaviours to preserve the vascular network. New approaches should be proposed, particularly focused on an integrated perspective and including the nephrologist and the dialysis nurse during pre-dialysis. This approach must be implemented through programmes enabling the continuous assessment of the development of self-care behaviours for the preservation of the vascular network.

Instrument to Assess Self-care With the Arteriovenous Fistula

Literature shows that a number of instruments can be used to collect information on patients' self-care behaviours with venous preservation. The Scale for Assessment of Self-Care Behaviours in Anticipation of Arteriovenous Fistula Creation (ASBAC-AVF) was proposed by Sousa et al., which enables the determination of self-care behaviours for the preservation of the vascular network of end-stage renal disease patients (Sousa et al. 2015b). It is based on Dorothea Orem's Self-Care Theory.

The scale consists of four items and shows good metrics in terms of test–retest reliability and internal consistency, with a Cronbach's alpha of 0.83. Its application is fast, it is self-administered, and it can be filled in by a healthcare professional when the patient has visual problems or an upper limb disability that prevents him/her from writing. The items are aimed at protecting the vascular network, preventing damage to the veins and trauma to the arms during pre-dialysis. Each item has a 5-point Likert scale, ranging from 1 (I never perform this self-care) to 5 (I always perform this self-care). The final score is given by the sum of all the items, ranging between 4 and 20. The higher the percentage, i.e., the closer to 100, the greater the frequency of self-care behaviours (Sousa et al. 2015b). The scale was adapted and validated in Brazil.

Its clinical use is limited to people with a proper cognitive condition and full memory.

Self-Care of the Arteriovenous Fistula During the Maturation Period

The maturation period of the AVF is the time between its construction and the first cannulation. Sousa (2012) defined two distinct moments in the AVF maturation period: the first 48 hours after construction and the maturation period. In the former period, i.e., 48 hours after construction, the patient should be trained to check the functionality of the AVF, detect problems with the distal hyperfusion, prevent infection, and carry out self-care behaviours for the preservation of the AVF (Table 1).

Promoting the development of the AVF during the maturation period is very important, with an increase in the diameter and the thickness of the vein wall. All the self-care behaviours usually carried out by the patient must be continued during this period and the patient should be trained how to identify the normal thrill and pulse as well.

Literature has shown the importance for the patient to carry out hand and full arm exercises, which can effectively improve blood flow in the drainage vein and in the brachial artery, upper arm strength and clinical maturation rate (Nantakool et al. 2020, 2022; Ribeiro et al. 2024). Exercises involving tightening a clothespin, squeezing a softball, biceps curl, handgrip exercises, dumbbells, and elastic bands aim to promote the development of the AVF vein (Chen et al. 2023; Ribeiro et al. 2024). This type of

Table 1 Self-care behaviours during the 48 hours after the creation of the AVF

Elevate the arm of the AVF to enhance circulation and reduce or prevent oedema; keeping the arm extended and well supported, avoiding all movements that favour haemorrhage or impair the venous return
Feel the thrill twice a day
Detect cooling of the distal extremities, numbness, tingling, and changes in the motor function of the hand
Protect the AVF arm from situations that could favour infection or damage the access
Detect signs and symptoms of infection with an AVF
Blood pressure cannot be assessed in the AVF arm
Avoid venipunctures in the AVF arm
Carrying heavy objects with the AVF arm should be avoided
Avoid positions that may hinder venous return (sleeping upon the AVF arm or its flexion)
The use of tight clothing should be avoided, and also avoid places with high temperature differences
Accessories (bracelets, watches, wristbands, gloves, and tight cuffs) that hinder venous return should be used with caution

exercise can be considered isotonic (exercise with joint movement and that applies a constant weight on the muscles) and isometric (exercise with muscle contraction but without any joint movement) (Nantakool et al. 2022).

A number of systematic reviews and meta-analyses show that more studies are required to draw a sound conclusion about the impact of maturation exercises on the AVF. A study involving 119 patients aged 20–80 years with wrist AVF were included in a basic handgrip exercises programme (group A), an advanced programme (group B), or an advanced plus upper arm banding programme (group C), found no significant differences in mean vessel diameter or blood flow 14, 30, 60, and 90 days after creation ($p = 0.55, 0.88, 0.21$, and 0.19 for diameter; $0.94, 0.81, 0.49$, and 0.56 for flow, respectively) (Chen et al. 2023). This finding is explained by the quality of such studies, the variability in the type of interventions used, and the small number of participants (Nantakool et al. 2020, 2022; Meng et al. 2024).

To the best of our knowledge, we are not aware of any studies assessing the frequency of self-care behaviours with the AVF carried out by patients during the maturation period. Such an assessment would lead to the identification of not only the behaviours carried out most often but also of those seldom or never performed. Further research is required in order to determine the frequency of self-care behaviours in HD patients which will enable the design and tuning of appropriate strategies.

Instrument for the Assessment of Self-care With the Arteriovenous Fistula

Instruments designed to assess self-care behaviours with the AVF during the maturation period are not available in the literature. Sousa (2014) introduced the Scale for Assessment of Self-Care Behaviours in the Period of Arteriovenous Fistula Maturation (ASBPM-AVF), but failed to provide the analysis of the construct (Sousa 2014).

This scale was based on Dorothea Orem's Self-Care Theory, and each item represents a different self-care behaviour with the purposes of keeping the AVF working and promoting the development of the drainage vein. Each item has a 5-point Likert scale, ranging from 1 (I never carry out this self-care) to 5 (I always carry out this self-care). Sousa has currently submitted a manuscript with the final version of the ASBPM-AVF (with a new sample). This instrument can be used by nephrology nurses to assess self-care behaviours with the AVF during the maturation period.

Self-Care With the Arteriovenous Fistula During Haemodialysis

Patients should carry out self-care behaviours with the AVF from the beginning of the haemodialysis treatment because its effectiveness can be affected by the access condition (Sousa et al. 2014). Furthermore, such behaviours should be continued in the maturation period and some new ones, specific to this period, should be added as well, focusing on intradialytic care, bruising, needle removal, and some aspects of interdialytic care (Table 2).

Different frequencies of self-care behaviours with the AVF performed by patients have been reported in the literature, ranging from 54.52% to 83.9% (Sousa et al.

Table 2 Self-care behaviours with the AVF during haemodialysis

Washing the arm before cannulation
Identifying signs and symptoms of dialysis-induced hypotension and informing the nurse
Gently moving the arm with the AVF during HD
Applying dynamic pressure during haemostasis
Applying ice for the first 24 hours after haematoma
Applying heparinoid ointment twice a day after 24 hours
Avoiding to apply heparinoid ointment on the day of HD
Removing the dressing of the cannulation site after 24 hours

2017, 2022; Bulbul et al. 2023; Şahan et al. 2023; Dilbilir and Kavurmaci 2024). Furthermore, some studies show inappropriate self-care behaviours with their access by 97.7% of patients (Pessoa and Linhares 2015). Therefore, it is clear that a large number of patients do not carry out the appropriate self-care behaviours and need training.

As reported by a number of studies, some self-care behaviours with the AVF are performed more often than others. On the one hand, those related to managing signs and symptoms are performed with an average frequency ranging from 20.9% to 94.8% (Sousa et al. 2017; Lira et al. 2021; Bulbul et al. 2023). They are associated with the identification of the signs and symptoms of dialysis-induced hypotension (headaches and cramps) and distal hyperfusion (wounds or lesions and pain in the hand). Patients should also acknowledge such signs and symptoms in order to warn the nurse when they return to the dialysis centre or during dialysis. Other behaviours should also be adopted, such as protecting the AVF arm from shocks or blows, or performing finger haemostasis at home if the cannulation sites are bleeding.

On the other hand, those behaviours related to the prevention of complications are carried out with an average frequency ranging from 33.5% to 77.4% (Sousa et al. 2017; Bulbul et al. 2023; Dilbilir and Kavurmaci 2024). They are related to the identification of functionality (feeling the motion) and signs of local infection, protection of the fistula arm from trauma and blood collection, caring for haematomas, and the identification of problems with distal hyperfusion.

Several studies have shown that the frequency of self-care behaviours associated with managing signs and symptoms is larger than that of behaviours related to preventing complications (Sousa et al. 2017; Lira et al. 2021), which may be caused by some previous problem or by changes in the condition of the fistula arm. Patients value self-care behaviours associated with existing problems in the fistula arm more than those that help the prevention of complications. These results prove the need for programmes designed to train patients on how to perform self-care behaviours with the AVF.

Literature shows that the frequency of fistula self-care behaviours can be negatively and positively affected by several variables (Sousa et al. 2017, 2022; Martins and Moura 2023; Alabacak and Arslan 2024). In a study of 89 HD patients with AVF, self-care behaviours were negatively affected by the patient's location (patients living in peripheral locations) (OR = 0.45, CI: 0.204–0.995) and positively by material status (widow) (OR = 7.4, CI: 2.051–26.445), education (6 years: OR = 3.3,

CI: 1.021–107.23; 9 years: OR = 4.4, CI: 1.435–13.753; 12 years: OR = 2.8, CI: 1.203–7.548), employment (retired) (OR = 4.1, CI: 1.703–10.006), AVF life span in months (OR = 1.007, CI: 1.0002, 1.015), and absence of complications with the AVF (OR = 2.6, CI: 1.079–6.202) (Sousa et al. 2022). Another study of 259 patients reported that those who did not have an income-generating job had higher self-care behaviours than those who worked (mean ± standard deviation: 67.36 ± 6.84 and 64.86 ± 6.27, $p > 0.05$, respectively) and also found that women had better self-care than men (67.45 ± 6.27 and 64.70 ± 6.84, $p > 0.05$, respectively) (Alabacak and Arslan 2024). However, a study of 216 HD patients showed that self-care behaviours can be positively influenced by higher levels of patient education (patients with a university education had better AVF self-care) (Bulbul et al. 2023).

Self-care behaviours associated with the management of signs and symptoms are negatively affected by the presence of a previous fistula (7.99, 95% CI: –14.78; 1.21) (Sousa et al. 2017), the training agent (when not a nephrologist or nephrology nurse) (Martins and Moura 2023) (29.78, 95% CI: –46.74; 12.82) (Sousa et al. 2017), patient's location (OR = 0.32, CI = 0.903–0.976) (Sousa et al. 2022), and level of education, $p > 0.05$ (Martins and Moura 2023). Furthermore, they are positively affected by the fistula life span (0.039, 95% CI: –0.003; 0.082) (Sousa et al. 2017).

Self-care behaviours associated with the prevention of complications are positively affected by gender (women have better self-care) (Martins and Moura 2023) (9.27, 95% CI: 2.77; 15.77) (Sousa et al. 2017), level of education (higher education, better self-care) (Martins and Moura 2023), marital status (widow) (OR = 3.9, CI: 1.184–13.150) (Sousa et al. 2022), employment (retired) (OR = 4.9, CI: 1.848–12.907) (Sousa et al. 2022), and hypertension (14.85, 95% CI: 4.49; 25.21) (Sousa et al. 2017). They are negatively affected by the training agent (when not a nephrologist or nephrology nurse) (26.23, 95% CI: –42.29; 10.17) (Sousa et al. 2017), age (OR = 0.94, CI: 0.903–0.976) (Sousa et al. 2022; Martins and Moura 2023), and marital status (single or divorced) (OR = 0.13, CI: 0.037–0.422) (Sousa et al. 2022).

A small number of studies address the relationship between health literacy and self-care with the vascular access. However, Bulbul et al. highlighted the relationship between literacy and fistula self-care behaviours. Patients with better literacy ($r = 0.421, p < 0.001$) have better AVF-related self-care behaviours (Bulbul et al. 2023).

Very few studies on the self-care profile of patients with AVF on HD are available in the literature. A single study with 101 patients identified two profiles, which were labelled moderate self-care and high self-care (Sousa et al. 2020). The "moderate self-care" profile mainly includes male patients, with higher education level, employed, with shorter dialysis vintage, with lower AVF duration, and whose information on AVF care is less often provided by the nephrologist. On the contrary, the "high self-care" profile mainly includes female patients, with lower education level, retired, with longer dialysis vintage, with higher AVF duration, and whose information on AVF care is more often provided by the nephrologist (Sousa et al. 2020).

Profiles of self-care with the AVF concern different levels of capacity, autonomy, and involvement of patients in the management of their own health. Such profiles are used to assess and understand the extent to which the patient is able to carry out self-care activities, considering their practical skills and knowledge of their own health condition. The profiles help to identify each patient's level of proficiency in carrying out the care required to prevent complications and manage signs and symptoms with the AVF. They are also important tools for nephrology nurses to provide personalized training according to the patient's needs and abilities. The existence of self-care profiles for patients with AVF can help directing both the patient and the nephrology nurse towards more effective and safer management according to their clinical condition.

Further studies are needed in order to determine the number of self-care profiles and their characteristics. Describing such characteristics makes the identification of the patient's needs and skills possible with the aim of offering specific support, from intensive support to encouraging autonomy and proactivity. The definition of those profiles can also help adjusting the length and intensity of training programmes designed to enhance patients' acquisition of self-care behaviours with the AVF.

Several guidelines have recommended the need to train patients with ESRD to carry out self-care behaviours with their AVF. There are different training methods available in the literature to improve such behaviours. The face-to-face training method is often used in this population (Sousa et al. 2021; Şahan et al. 2023), as well as group training (Sousa et al. 2021; Dilbilir and Kavurmaci 2024). Literature shows that printed materials (Dilbilir and Kavurmaci 2024), videos, and audiovisual tools (Şahan et al. 2023; Pessoa et al. 2024) can also be used as educational methods that can be used separately or together.

A quasi-experimental study involving 89 patients with AVF undergoing HD (41 and 48 patients in the control and intervention groups, respectively) found that the intervention group showed significant improvements in overall self-care behaviours, in managing signs and symptoms, and in preventing complications after the intervention (79.2–91.4%, $p < 0.001$; 90.1–94.4%, $p = 0.004$; and from 72.7–89.5%, $p < 0.001$, respectively) (Sousa et al. 2021). These authors designed a Structured Intervention for Self-Care with the AVF, consisting of both a theoretical and a practical part, with the aim of identifying the signs/symptoms or situations that can compromise the proper functioning of an AVF (Sousa et al. 2021).

The theoretical part comprised six presentations held in an appropriate room over 2 days before patients started HD treatment. Each presentation had a maximum of eight patients and lasted 30 minutes, based on the group training method. The practical part began 1 week after the theoretical part and lasted 2 weeks. Each participant had two individual 15-minute sessions designed from the simulation-based learning (Sousa et al. 2021).

A controlled, randomized experimental study was carried out involving 60 patients with AVF (30 patients in both the control and the experimental groups) using the video as educational method (Şahan et al. 2023). The video session lasted 20 minutes and began after an hour of HD, using the bedside television. Patients watched the video twice a week, with a break of 1 week. Both groups were evaluated at two and four weeks post-intervention. At both time points the experimental group showed a significant improvement compared control group in the development of self-care behaviours (63.06–71.40%, $p = 0.000$, and 63.63–73.16%, $p = 0.000$, respectively) (Şahan et al. 2023).

In 2024, another study showed the positive impact of this method on patients' self-care behaviours with the AVF (Pessoa et al. 2024). In this randomized controlled trial with 55 patients (27 and 28 in the control and in the intervention groups, respectively), the experimental group watched an educational video lasting 3 minutes and 17 seconds during the first hour of HD (Pessoa et al. 2024). This educational technology had a positive effect on the self-care of patients with AVF at 7 and 14 days after the intervention ($p = 0.004$ and $p < 0.001$, respectively) (Pessoa et al. 2024).

Printed materials can be used as another method of educating AVF patients to promote their self-care behaviours with the access. A randomized controlled trial with 66 patients analysed the effect of AVF care training given to HD patients using written educational materials on patients' self-care behaviours (Dilbilir and Kavurmaci 2024). Such materials consisted of a book with different topics, organized by week and lasting 4 weeks (each topic corresponded to 1 week). Patients in the experimental group had a significant increase in their self-care behaviours (54.52%–73.77%, $p < 0.001$) unlike those in the control group (56.14%–58.24%, $p = 0.115$) (Dilbilir and Kavurmaci 2024).

Educational methods are appropriate tools to improve self-care behaviours in HD patients with an AVF. However, further studies are required to assess the effect of these and other methods (such as educational games and gamification, simulation-based learning, practical workshops, motivational counselling, experience-based teaching) on the acquisition of self-care behaviours by patients.

The choice of educational method depends on the patient's profile (age, education level, preferences, and health conditions), the goal of education (information delivery, skill practice, or behaviour change), and available resources (time, budget, and access to technology). Combining different methods is often a more effective strategy for providing comprehensive and rigorous education.

Instrument to Assess Self-care With the Arteriovenous Fistula

A few instruments have been introduced to be used in clinical practice with the purpose of identifying self-care behaviours by patients on HD. The Assessment Scale for Self-Care Behaviours with Arteriovenous Fistula in Haemodialysis (ASBHD-AVF) is the most widely used scale to determine the frequency of self-care behaviours by patients with these conditions (Sousa et al. 2015a).

The ASBHD-AVF is made up of 16 items, with a two-dimensional structure: the first, called Prevention of Complications, with 10 items, assesses self-care behaviours that should be carried out to prevent infection and thrombosis of the fistula; the second, called management of signs and symptoms, with six items, evaluates self-care behaviours aimed at the signs and symptoms of complications with the access (Sousa et al. 2015a). The ASBHD-AVF showed good metrics in the original study, both in terms of test–retest reliability and internal consistency, with the Cronbach's alpha being 0.8, 0.72, and 0.8 for the overall scale, the Prevention of Complications, and the Management of Signs and Symptoms subscales, respectively. Each item has a 5-point Likert scale, ranging from 1 (never performs this self-care) to 5 (always performs this self-care) (Sousa et al. 2015a). The final score is found by adding up all the items, ranging from 16 to 80. The numerical value of the final score is used to compute the frequency of self-care behaviours carried out by the patient with the fistula. Higher percentages (closer to 100) mean a higher frequency of fistula self-care behaviours.

The ASBHD-AVF has been validated in China (Yang et al. 2019), Turkey (İkiz et al. 2021), Brazil (Lira et al. 2021), Morocco (Loubna et al. 2025), and Iran (Sharif-Nia et al. 2024), and is currently in the final process of validation in Taiwan, Austalia, Spain and Colombia.

This scale is short, easy, and quick to apply (15 minutes are usually enough), is self-administered, and can be filled in by the healthcare professional if the patient has visual problems or an upper limb disability preventing him/her from writing. However, its clinical use is restricted to people with appropriate cognitive condition and full memory.

2 Practical Implications

AVF care is very important to enhance access patency. Patients should be trained to develop self-care behaviours in order to detect situations that may compromise their access, preserve the vascular network, monitor access functionality, and prevent infection and thrombosis. Nephrology nurses should design educational strategies and methods in order to improve the acquisition of AVF self-care behaviours.

References

Alabacak Ş, Arslan S (2024) The relationship between self-care behaviours regarding arteriovenous fistula and the fear of fistula failure in individuals receiving haemodialysis treatment. J Res Nurs 29(4–5):388–398

Allen A, Megargell J, Brown D, Lynch F, Singh H, Singh Y et al (2000) Venous thrombosis associated with the placement of peripherally inserted central catheters. J Vasc Interv Radiol 11(10):1309–1314

Bulbul E, Yildiz Ayvaz M, Yeni T, Turen S, Efil S (2023) Arteriovenous fistula self-care behaviors in patients receiving hemodialysis treatment: association with health literacy and self-care agency. J Vasc Access 24(6):1358–1364

Chen J, Fu H, Hii I, Tseng H, Chang P, Chang C et al (2023) A randomized trial of postoperative handgrip exercises for fistula maturation in patients with newly created wrist radiocephalic arteriovenous fistulas. Kidney Int Rep 8(3):566–574.

Dilbilir Y, Kavurmaci M (2024) Determining the effect of arteriovenous fistula care training on the self-care behaviors of hemodialysis patients. Ther Apher Dial 28(6):893–903

Hakim R, Himmelfarb J (2009) Hemodialysis access failure: a call to action - revisited. Kidney Int 76(10):1040–1048

İkiz S, Usta Y, Sousa C, Dias V, Magalhães A, Lins S et al (2021) Validation of the scale of assessment of self-care behaviours for arteriovenous fistula in patients ongoing haemodialysis in Turkey. J Ren Care 47(4):279–284

Lira M, Sousa C, Wanderley M, Pessoa N, Lemos K, Manzini C et al (2021) Scale of assessment of self-care behaviors with arteriovenous fistula in hemodialysis: a psychometric study in Brazil. Clin Nurs Res 30(6):875–882

Loubna M, Abdelhafid B, Mounia A, Sousa C, Mohamed C (2025) Moroccan adaptation of the 'self-care behaviour assessment scale' for arteriovenous fistula in haemodialysis. J Ren Care 51(1):e70004. https://doi.org/10.1111/jorc.70004

Martins M, Moura S (2023) Analysis of self-care behaviors in patients with arteriovenous fistula. Rev Enf Ref 6(2):e29211. https://doi.org/10.12707/RVI23.11.29211

Meng L, Zhang T, Ho P (2024) Effect of exercises on the maturation of newly created arteriovenous fistulas over distal and proximal upper limb: a systematic review and meta-analysis. J Vasc Access 25(1):40–50

Nantakool S, Rerkasem K, Reanpang T, Worraphan S, Prasannarong M (2020) A systematic review with meta-analysis of the effects of arm exercise training programs on arteriovenous fistula maturation among people with chronic kidney disease. Hemodial Int 24(4):439–453

Nantakool S, Reanpang T, Prasannarong M, Pongtam S, Rerkasem K (2022) Upper limb exercise for arteriovenous fistula maturation in people requiring permanent haemodialysis access. Cochrane Database Syst Rev 10(10):CD013327

Pessoa N, Linhares F (2015) Hemodialysis patients with arteriovenous fistula: knowledge, attitude and practice. Esc Anna Nery 19(1):73–79

Pessoa N, Lima L, Santos G, Frazão C, Sousa C, Ramos V (2020) Self-care actions for the maintenance of the arteriovenous fistula: an integrative review. Int J Nurs Sci 7(3):369–377

Pessoa N, Sales J, Sousa C,LM, Frazão C, Ramos V (2024) Educational video for self-care with arteriovenous fistula in renal patients: randomized clinical trial. Rev Lat Am Enfermagem 17(32):e4185

Ribeiro H, Duarte M, Andrade F, Sousa M, Baiao V, Monteiro J et al (2024) Exercise guide to help on arteriovenous fistula maturation and maintenance. J Vasc Access 25(1):318–322

Şahan S, Yıldız A, Özdemir C, İsmailoğlu E (2023) The effect of video-based fistula care education on hemodialysis patients' self-care behaviors: a randomized controlled study. Ther Apher Dial 27(6):1095–1102

Sharif-Nia H, Farhadi B, Mazhari S, Sousa C, Taebi M, Hoseinzadeh E et al (2024) Validity and reliability of the Persian version of the scale of the assessment of self-care behaviors with arteriovenous fistula in patients on hemodialysis. J Nurs Meas JNM-2024-0080.R1. https://doi.org/10.1891/JNM-2024-0080

Sousa C (2012) Caring for the person arteriovenous fistula: model for continuous improvement. Rev Port Sau Pub 30(1):11–17

Sousa C (2014) Caring for people with end-stage renal disease with an arteriovenous fistula. Ph.D. Dissertation submitted to the Abel Salazar Institute of Biomedical Sciences of the University of Porto

Sousa C, Apóstolo J, Figueiredo M, Martins M, Dias V (2014) Interventions to promote self-care of people with arteriovenous fistula. J Clin Nurs 23(13–14):1796–1802

Sousa C, Apóstolo J, Figueiredo M, Dias V, Teles P, Martins M (2015a) Construction and validation of a scale of assessment of self-care behaviors with arteriovenous fistula in hemodialysis. Hemodial Int 19(2):306–313

Sousa C, Figueiredo M, Dias V, Teles P, Apóstolo J (2015b) Construction and validation of a scale of assessment of self-care behaviours anticipatory to creation of arteriovenous fistula. J Clin Nurs 24(23–24):3674–3680.

Sousa C, Marujo P, Teles P, Lira M, Novais M (2017) Self-care on hemodialysis: behaviors with the arteriovenous fistula. Ther Apher Dial 21(2):195–199

Sousa C, Ligeiro I, Teles P, Paixão L, Dias V, Cristovão A (2018) Self-care in preserving the vascular network: old problem, new challenge for the medical staff. Ther Apher Dial 22(4):332–336

Sousa C, Marujo P, Teles P, Lira M, Dias V, Novais M (2020) Self-care behavior profiles with arteriovenous fistula in hemodialysis patients. Clin Nurs Res 29(6):363–367

Sousa C, Paquete A, Teles P, Pinto C, Dias V, Ribeiro O et al (2021) Investigating the effect of a structured intervention on the development of self-care behaviors with arteriovenous fistula in hemodialysis patients. Clin Nurs Res 30(6):866–874

Sousa C, Teles P, Paquete A, Dias V, Manzini C, Nicole A et al (2022) Effects of demographic and clinical character on differences in self-care behavior levels with arteriovenous fistula by hemodialysis patients: an ordinal logistic regression approach. Ther Apher Dial 26(5):992–998 van der Veer S, Haller M, Pittens C, Broerse J, Castledine C, Gallieni M et al (2015) Setting priorities for optimizing vascular access decision making – an international survey of patients and clinicians. PLoS One 10(7):1–13

Yang M, Zhao H, Ding X, Zhu G, Yang Z, Ding L et al (2019) Self-care behavior of hemodialysis patients with arteriovenous fistula in China: a multicenter, cross-sectional study. Ther Apher Dial 23(2):167–172

GPSR Compliance

The European Union's (EU) General Product Safety Regulation (GPSR) is a set of rules that requires consumer products to be safe and our obligations to ensure this.

If you have any concerns about our products, you can contact us on ProductSafety@springernature.com

In case Publisher is established outside the EU, the EU authorized representative is:

Springer Nature Customer Service Center GmbH
Europaplatz 3
69115 Heidelberg, Germany

Batch number: 09456952

Printed by Printforce, the Netherlands